PRESS HERE!

AYURVEDIC HEAD MASSAGE
~ FOR BEGINNERS ~

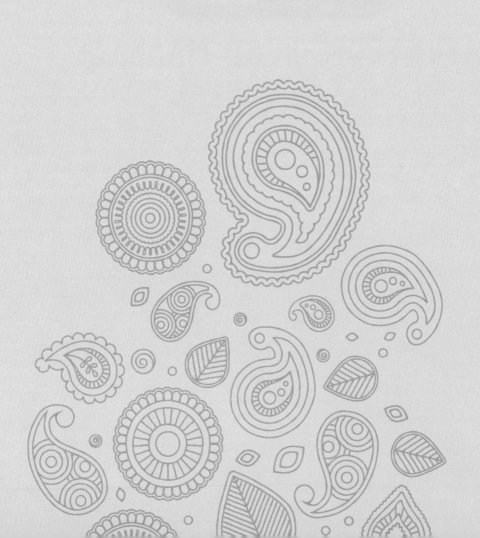

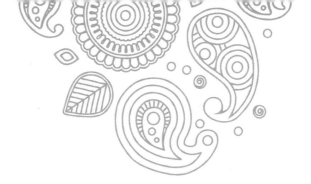

PRESS HERE!

AYURVEDIC HEAD MASSAGE
~ FOR BEGINNERS ~

A PRACTICE FOR OVERALL HEALTH AND WELLNESS

HILLARY ARRIETA

Illustrations by
Emily Portnoi

FAIR WINDS

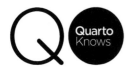

Inspiring | Educating | Creating | Entertaining

Brimming with creative inspiration, how-to projects, and useful information to enrich your everyday life, Quarto Knows is a favorite destination for those pursuing their interests and passions. Visit our site and dig deeper with our books into your area of interest: Quarto Creates, Quarto Cooks, Quarto Homes, Quarto Lives, Quarto Drives, Quarto Explores, Quarto Gifts, or Quarto Kids.

First Published in 2021 by Fair Winds Press,
an imprint of The Quarto Group.
100 Cummings Center, Suite 265-D,
Beverly, MA 01915, USA.
T (978) 282-9590 F (978) 283-2742

Fair Winds Press titles are also available at discount for retail, wholesale, promotional, and bulk purchase. For details, contact the Special Sales Manager by email at specialsales@quarto.com or by mail at The Quarto Group, Attn: Special Sales Manager, 100 Cummings Center, Suite 265-D, Beverly, MA 01915, USA.

25 24 23 22 21 1 2 3 4 5

ISBN: 978-1-58923-978-4

Digital edition published in 2021

QUAR.336361

Conceived, edited, and designed by Quarto Publishing,
an imprint of The Quarto Group,
The Old Brewery, 6 Blundell Street,
London N7 9BH, United Kingdom

Editor: Claire Waite Brown
Designer and Illustrator: Emily Portnoi
Art Director: Gemma Wilson
Publisher: Samantha Warrington

Printed in Singapore

The information in this book is for educational purposes only. It is not intended to replace the advice of a physician or medical practitioner. Please see your health-care provider before beginning any new health program.

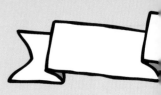

Chapter 1
BASIC PRINCIPLES   10

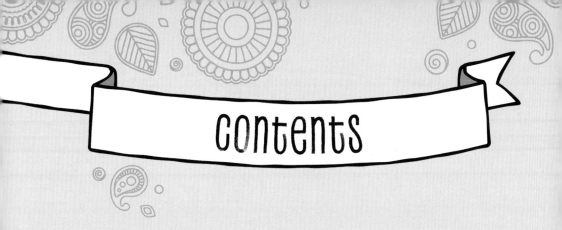

Contents

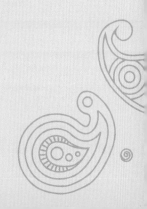

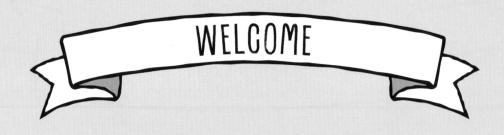

WELCOME

THERAPEUTIC MASSAGE FOUND ITS WAY INTO MY LIFE IN MY EARLY TWENTIES AS I SEARCHED FOR A PEACEFUL LIFESTYLE AND CAREER TO HELP MANAGE THE SYMPTOMS OF AN ANXIETY CONDITION THAT HAD STARTED TO PUT A STRAIN ON MY EVERYDAY LIFE. I TOOK A FRONT DESK JOB AT A HIGH-END DAY SPA, WHERE I MET SEVERAL MASSAGE THERAPISTS WHO ENCOURAGED ME TO LOOK INTO MASSAGE SCHOOLS. I AM SO GLAD I DID. MASSAGE SCHOOL WAS THE PERFECT FIT FOR ME, AND I LOVED EVERYTHING ABOUT IT.

AS I DUG DEEPER INTO MY STUDIES, I DISCOVERED THAT EASTERN MASSAGE TECHNIQUES AND THEORY PULLED AT MY HEART, AND BEING ABLE TO CARE FOR OTHERS IN SUCH A PRECISE WAY WITHIN THE FRAMEWORK AYURVEDA PROVIDES, INSPIRES THE PITTA IN ME—YOU'LL LEARN MORE ABOUT THAT LATER!

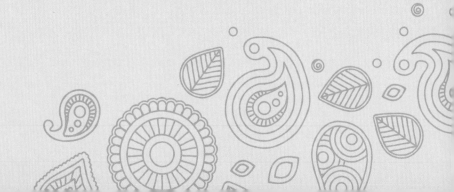

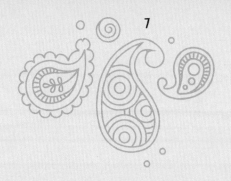

THE BEAUTY IN RITUAL-STYLE BODYWORK AND OTHER OLD-WORLD HEALING SYSTEMS LIKE AYURVEDA IS PROFOUND. WORKING WITH OTHERS TOWARD WELLNESS GIVES ME A SENSE OF "BEING IN THE FLOW." I LOVE CREATING A HAVEN AWAY FROM THE BUSY WORLD, AND FOR ME, IT CONTINUES TO BE AN HONOR TO DO THIS TYPE OF WORK.

I BELIEVE THAT IT'S HARD TO THRIVE WHEN WE'RE STUCK IN A LIFESTYLE THAT DOESN'T ALLOW FOR REST, A VITAL PART OF STAYING WELL. BY SHARING AYURVEDIC HEAD MASSAGE WITH YOU IN THIS BOOK, I HOPE TO INSPIRE YOU AND GIVE YOU TOOLS TO CREATE A SENSE OF PEACE IN YOUR EVERYDAY LIFE AND THE LIVES OF YOUR FRIENDS AND FAMILY.

Hillary Arrieta

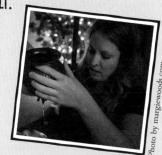

Photo by margiewoods.com

DISCLAIMER

The information shared in this book is not a substitute for professional massage therapy education.

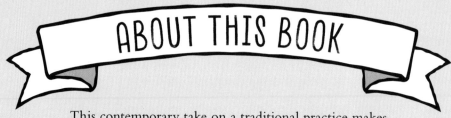

ABOUT THIS BOOK

This contemporary take on a traditional practice makes Ayurvedic head massage accessible to all, whether you are treating yourself, a friend or a family member.

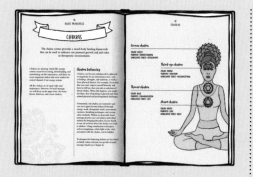

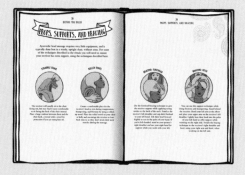

Chapter 1
BASIC PRINCIPLES
PAGES 10-21

In this chapter you will learn what Ayurvedic head massage is and how it can help you, and find out about the principles of doshas, chakras, and marmas.

Chapter 2
BEFORE YOU BEGIN
PAGES 22-31

Before you begin you will take a few steps to prepare your space, yourself, and, where relevant, your massage receiver. This chapter also looks at the various strokes you will be using in your massages.

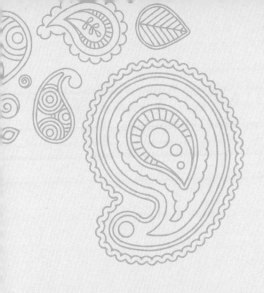

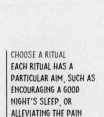

CHOOSE A RITUAL
EACH RITUAL HAS A
PARTICULAR AIM, SUCH AS
ENCOURAGING A GOOD
NIGHT'S SLEEP, OR
ALLEVIATING THE PAIN
OF A HEADACHE.

STEP-BY-STEP
CLEAR TEXT AND
VISUALS GUIDE
YOU THROUGH THE
MASSAGE ROUTINE.

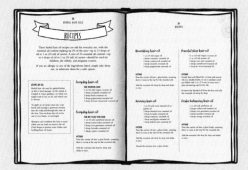

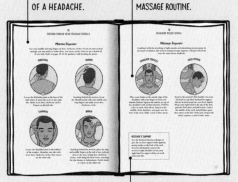

TIPS
ALONG THE WAY THERE ARE TIPS
TO HELP YOU KEEP YOURSELF
AND, WHERE RELEVANT, YOUR
RECEIVER, COMFORTABLE.

Chapter 3
HERBAL HAIR OILS
PAGES 32-39

I have created herbal oil mixes designed
specifically to be used with the rituals
described in Chapter 4, should you want to.
Learn how to make them here, and discover
the ingredients you can use to make your
own herbal hair oils.

Chapter 4
FOCUSED INDIAN HEAD MASSAGE RITUALS
PAGES 40-125

This chapter contains eight massage routines
designed to address particular areas of concern
or for general wellbeing. Follow the step-by-step
instructions to massage yourself or a partner.
Use regularly to feel physically, spiritually, and
mentally nourished.

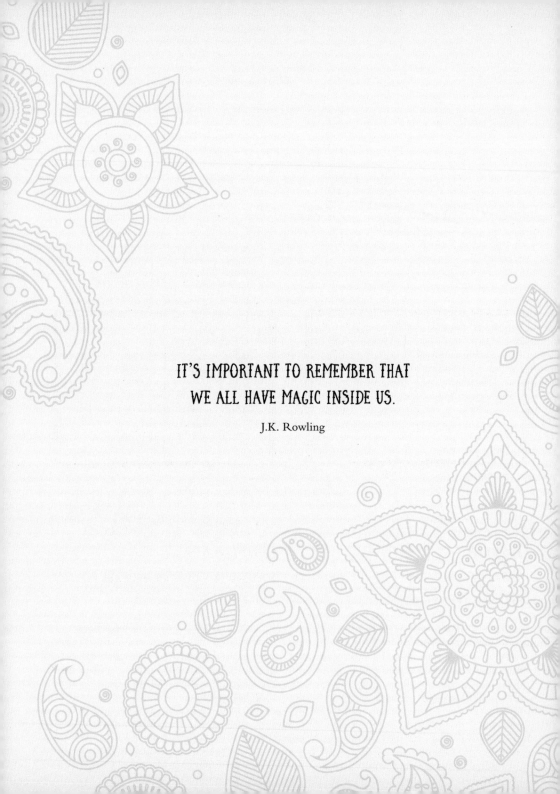

IT'S IMPORTANT TO REMEMBER THAT
WE ALL HAVE MAGIC INSIDE US.

J.K. Rowling

BASIC PRINCIPLES

This chapter looks at the history and practice of
Ayurvedic head massage, including an introduction
to doshas, chakras, and marmas.

WHAT IS AYURVEDIC HEAD MASSAGE?

Ayurveda, originating from India, is one of the planet's oldest healing systems, and Indian head massage—also known as champissage— is a form of Ayurvedic therapy.

The benefits of an Ayurvedic head massage are extensive, and effective physically, mentally, and emotionally. There are also benefits for appearance and overall well-being.

Traditionally, women of the family practiced champissage to soothe headaches and other ailments, and to beautify their hair. The practice extended out into the skills of many Indian barbers and haircare professionals.

Modern-day Ayurvedic head massage

The techniques of Ayurvedic head massage that are practiced today were initially developed by Narendra Mehta, an Indian man who came to London in the late 1970s to study physical therapy. He was completely blind, and as a result, had developed a heightened sense of touch.

While in London he often reminisced about the head massages he received in India as a child. Mehta saw an opportunity to introduce and expand the art and culture of Indian head massage to the Western world, so founded the London Centre of Indian Champissage and began teaching his technique in 1995.

Mehta's version of Indian head massage focuses on more than just the head. It includes chakra balancing as well as massage techniques for the upper back, shoulders, upper arms, neck, face, and ears as well as the scalp.

Fusion

Since Mehta first introduced Indian head massage to the West, many new techniques have been created and adapted by other massage therapists. In this book, you'll find traditional Indian head massage techniques as taught by Mr Mehta, with the addition of Tibetan acupressure (using marma points), hair oil recipes, stretches, and yogic breathing practices.

Healthy body

Physically, an Ayurvedic head massage can ease restlessness and difficulties with sleeping. It helps reduce stress and relieves muscular tension, headaches, and eye strain. It can release tension that builds up in the neck and shoulders due to poor posture or physical or emotional stress.

Healthy mind

Mental and spiritual benefits from receiving a head massage include an increased sense of human connection between the giver and receiver. It can bring about a meditative mood that encourages relief from mild depression, burnout, and emotional overload.

Healthy hair

The women of India were onto something when they practiced head massage to enhance the beauty of their locks. Beauty benefits include improvement in the condition of the scalp and hair by exfoliating away dead skin and increasing local blood circulation. Massage provides nutrients to the living cells of the hair, giving it a luxurious appearance, while the use of nourishing, herbally infused oils can further increase the positive results of a beauty routine.

CAUTIONS AND CONTRAINDICATIONS

All massage therapy is generally considered non-invasive and safe. That said, there are a few circumstances when you should not receive a head massage, and massaging someone who's experiencing any of these conditions may cause an adverse reaction.

- Active skin disorders or infections of the scalp, such as weeping eczema, warts, boils, psoriasis, and acne
- Recent surgeries to the upper body
- Bruising to the upper body
- Acute swelling
- Inflamed skin, joints, or lymph nodes
- An active migraine
- Arthritis of the cervical spine
- Recent injury to the head or neck, such as whiplash or concussion
- A history of blood clots
- Uncontrolled high blood pressure

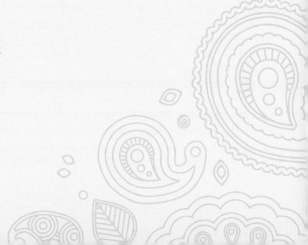

DOSHAS

In Ayurvedic theory, all humans embody a unique combination of the five elements: air, water, fire, earth, and space. These elements combine to form three energies, or doshas, described as Vata, Kapha, and Pitta.

Vata

Vata is the subtle energy responsible for movement in the body.

ELEMENTS
Air and space

PHYSICAL ASSOCIATIONS
Large intestine, bones, skin, ears, pelvis, and thighs.

PERSONALITY
People with Vata as their dominant dosha are quick-thinking, lean, and fast.

SUSCEPTIBILITY
May be susceptible to conditions such as anxiety, dry skin, and constipation.

Pitta

Pitta is the subtle energy responsible for metabolic body processes.

ELEMENTS
Fire and water

PHYSICAL ASSOCIATIONS
Small intestine, stomach, sweat glands, skin, eyes, and blood.

PERSONALITY
People with Pitta as their dominant dosha may have passionate personalities.

SUSCEPTIBILITY
Can experience sensitive/reactive skin and may be susceptible to conditions such as heart disease, stomach ulcers, inflammation, heartburn, and arthritis.

Kapha

Kapha is the subtle energy responsible for integrity, growth, repair, and moisture within the body.

ELEMENTS
Water and earth

PHYSICAL ASSOCIATIONS
Chest, lungs, and spinal fluid

PERSONALITY
People with Kapha as their dominant dosha are usually very calm.

SUSCEPTIBILITY
May be susceptible to conditions such as gallbladder problems, diabetes, obesity, and congestion.

The balance of a person's doshas may explain some of their qualities and individual preferences. An imbalanced combination of doshas, whether it is excessive or deficient, may cut off the natural flow of energy and increase the likelihood of experiencing certain illnesses. We all have traits from each dosha, but most people have a dominant, secondary, and least dominant dosha type. Discover your unique combination with this questionnaire.

On a sheet of paper, make a note of the statements in each list that best describe your true nature, then add up your answers to establish which trait you exhibit most of and least of, and the one in between.

Vata dosha	Pitta dosha	Kapha dosha
I have a slim, small build.	I have an athletic, medium build.	I have a sturdy, large build.
I have expressive eyes.	I have an intense gaze.	I have a soft gaze.
I am talkative.	I tend to ask precise questions.	I tend to be the strong, silent type.
I feel energized by the sun.	I love being in nature.	I prefer temperate climates.
I spend money easily.	I buy only the best.	I save money easily.
I am creative.	I take risks and am brave.	I am strong and caring.
I tend to have dry skin.	I tend to have sensitive, reactive skin.	I tend to have oily, smooth skin.
I'm a light sleeper.	I'm a good sleeper.	I'm a deep sleeper.
I tend to worry when I'm stressed.	I tend to be irritable when I'm stressed.	I tend to avoid people and responsibilities when I'm stressed.
I tend to lose weight unintentionally.	I can easily gain and/or lose weight.	It's hard for me to lose weight and I gain it easily.
TOTAL:	TOTAL:	TOTAL:

DOMINANT TYPE: SECONDARY TYPE: LEAST DOMINANT TYPE:

CHAKRAS

The chakra system provides a mind-body healing framework that can be used to enhance our personal growth and add value in therapeutic environments.

Chakras are spinning, wheel-like energy centers meant for receiving, downloading, and assimilating our life experiences, and there are seven important chakras that exist within the central channel of our energy system.

All the chakras are of equal value and importance. However, for head massage, we will focus on the upper four: the heart, throat, third-eye, and crown chakras.

Chakra balancing

Chakras can become unbalanced by upheaval or negativity in our internal processes, such as feelings, thoughts, and emotions, as well as from physical diseases. For example, if you feel that you can't express yourself honestly and have to tell lies, then you risk an unbalanced throat chakra. When this happens, you might develop a fear of speaking in general and other related physical and psychospiritual challenges.

Fortunately, our chakras are responsive and can once again become balanced through energy work, therapeutic touch, movements, exercises, breathing techniques, and various other methods. Within an Ayurvedic head massage practice you can balance individual chakras by bringing the palms of your hands to rest on or hover above the chakra you wish to address. Using visualization techniques, such as imagining a white light or the color associated with the chakra, can be helpful.

Techniques for balancing chakras are described in detail, where relevant, for specific focused massage rituals (see Chapter 4).

Crown chakra

COLOR: VIOLET
PURPOSE: UNDERSTANDING
UNBALANCE FORCE: ATTACHMENT

Third-eye chakra

COLOR: INDIGO
PURPOSE: INTUITION
UNBALANCE FORCE: MISCONCEPTION

Throat chakra

COLOR: BLUE
PURPOSE: COMMUNICATION
UNBALANCE FORCE: LIES

Heart chakra

COLOR: GREEN
PURPOSE: LOVE
UNBALANCE FORCE: GRIEF

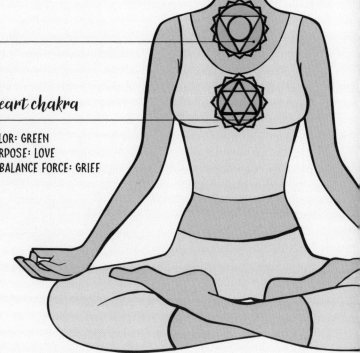

MARMAS

In Ayurvedic massage, marmas are pressure points located at the meeting places of ligaments, vessels, muscles, bones, and joints. They carry vital energy, which helps achieve balance within the doshas (see pages 14–15). By making gentle, circular movements on a marma point, the excess energy can be released and eliminated, helping to maintain balance through the doshas.

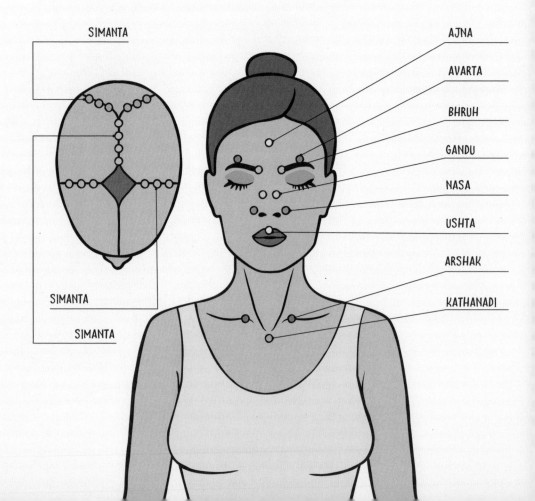

SIMANTA

SIMANTA

SIMANTA

AJNA

AVARTA

BHRUH

GANDU

NASA

USHTA

ARSHAK

KATHANADI

The wheres and whys of marma points

There are 107 marmas in total, 37 of which are in the head and neck.
In Chapter 4, we concentrate on 16 of these to enhance your massage
experience. Use the following guidelines to help you locate the points,
and to better understand why we massage them.

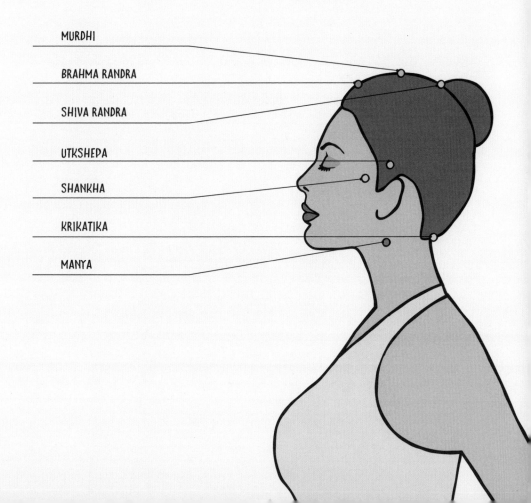

MURDHI

BRAHMA RANDRA

SHIVA RANDRA

UTKSHEPA

SHANKHA

KRIKATIKA

MANYA

MARMA POINT	LOCATION	PURPOSE
Ajna	The third-eye point, located about ½ inch (12mm) above the eyebrows in the center of the forehead.	Balances the body and mind. Enhances feelings of peace and equanimity.
Arshak	Located at the medial collarbone, close to the muscle that binds the skull to the sternum and clavicle.	Helps stimulate lymphatic drainage. Supports a clear complexion.
Avarta	Found in the middle of each eyebrow.	Enhances feelings of awareness. Soothes Vata energy.
Bhruh	Located on the upper orbital bone of the eyes.	Helps relieve eye strain and migraine pain.
Brahma Randra	Eight finger-widths above the eyebrows on the midline of the skull.	Eases insomnia or irregular sleep. Regulates body weight. May help balance hormonal functions.
Gandu	Located bilaterally halfway up the nose.	Drains extra fluid from the eye area.
Kathanadi	The hollow top of the sternum on each side.	Enhances circulation to the face. Clears congestion. Supports the health of the throat.
Kirkatika	Bilaterally located on either side of the spine where it meets the skull.	Eases tension in the neck and upper back. Improves hearing.
Manya	Bilaterally located on the side of the neck, four finger-widths below the ears.	Relieves congestion. Improves complexion. Supports fluid balance.

MARMA POINT	LOCATION	PURPOSE
Murdhi	To locate this point, bring the heel of your hand to the bridge of your nose. Allow your hand to relax over your forehead and fingers on the top of your head. Use your other hand to measure three finger-widths back from the middle finger.	Brings relaxation to the entire body. Eases neck and back tension. Promotes restful sleep. Supports blood circulation.
Nasa	Where the flares of the nostrils connect to the face on each side.	Helps enhance the clarity of the mind. May improve breathing.
Shankha	In the hollow points of each temple.	Calming and nourishing. Enhances memory. Encourages introspection.
Shiva Randra	Find this point by placing the heel of your hand in the center of your forehead on the hairline. Rest your hand over the top of your head and find the point at the tip of your middle finger.	May help regulate blood pressure. Helps memory.
Simanta	A number of random points along the sutures on the summit of the skull.	Improves the quality of relaxation. Eases tension in the scalp. Associated with the crown chakra
Ushta	Center of the upper lip.	Supports concentration. Supports relaxation.
Utkshepa	On the temporal arteries above each ear.	Calms the mind. Soothes Vata energy.

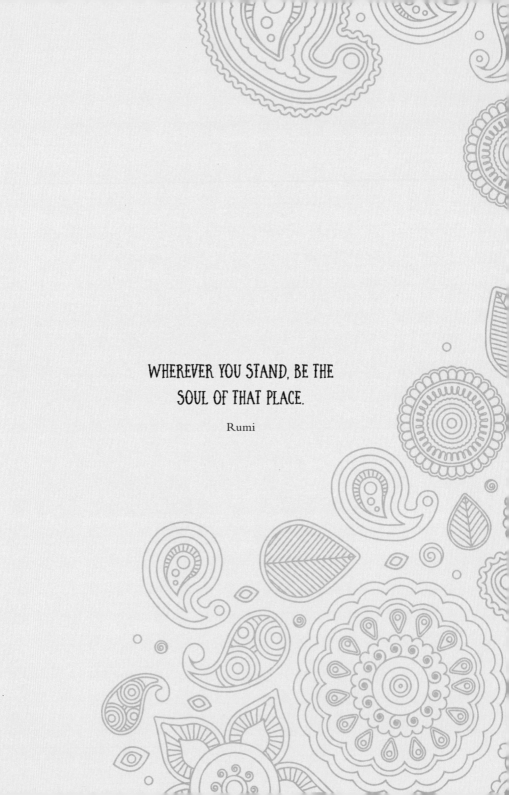

WHEREVER YOU STAND, BE THE
SOUL OF THAT PLACE.

Rumi

CHAPTER 2

BEFORE YOU BEGIN

This chapter considers the plans you may need to make before giving an Ayurvedic head massage, in order to prepare your space and yourself. You will learn about the various types of strokes used in a head massage, and ways to make the giver and receiver most comfortable.

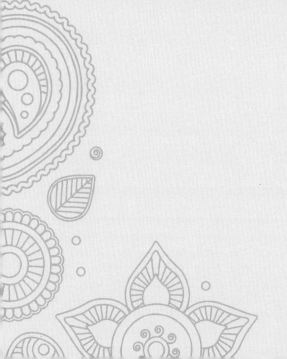

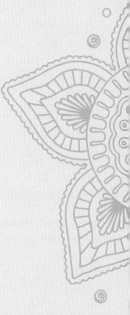

PRACTICAL PREPARATIONS

Make sure you have everything prepared before you begin a head massage ritual. Whether you are giving care to yourself or caring for others, the receiver should be comfortable and relaxed, and the provider, in the right frame of mind.

A good time

Choose a time when you will be completely free from distractions and can commit to relaxation and focus.

A good place

You will need a sturdy, upright chair without arms, positioned in an uncluttered space. You want the space to be clean and organized, and free from distractions.

Have some extra cushions on hand, since you might need to raise the receiver's seated position for your own comfort while massaging, and a large towel to use as a neck support (see page 28).

The space will need to be warm, which may mean employing an additional heat source during the colder months, or an electric fan for hotter climates.

The lighting should be calm and cozy, so dim the lights if you can or use lamps. You might also choose to play soothing music.

Personal considerations

Wear clean clothes with short sleeves and comfortable shoes, and avoid wearing any heavy perfumes or scents. If you have long hair, tie it back to keep it out of the way.

Make sure you breath is fresh, and trim and file your fingernails to avoid accidentally scratching the receiver—even if that is yourself! Remove your rings, watches, and bracelets, and wash your hands before and after each massage.

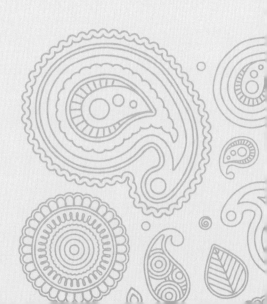

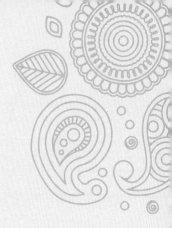

Supplies at the ready

If you are using one of my herbal hair oils (see pages 38–39), make sure you have it close at hand. Here's a handy list of other supplies you might choose to use:

- Large towel or blanket to protect the floor
- Hand sanitizer to use before you start
- Another large towel, or hairdressing cape, to protect the receiver's clothing
- An apron to protect the giver's clothing
- Essential oils and an aromatherapy diffuser
- A butterfly hair clip to pin back long hair
- Microfiber hair towel or shower cap for after the ritual
- Paper towels
- Clock

SEASONAL GUIDELINES

The changing seasons have an effect on our bodies, which might guide your choice of products. For example, winter months may cause the scalp and hair to dry, and therefore benefit from the use of herbal hair oils, while summer months might make the scalp more oily, in which case using oils is not desired.

You can also be influenced by the seasons in your preparations, for example by using seasonal smells, flowers, and plants in your environment. Choosing the right product for the time of the year is sure to give you or your partner a customized experience.

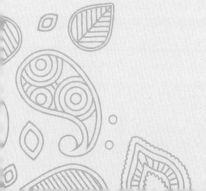

PREPARING YOUR BODY AND MIND

Begin each head massage treatment by setting the intention that your ritual is to serve the highest good of the receiver. Always give the receiver your undivided attention, and avoid any distractions during the massage. If you are massaging yourself, the same rules apply. Focus your attention on your goal for the session.

The exercises detailed can be used to focus your mind, wake up your muscles, release tension, and prevent against injury.

GROUND AND CENTER

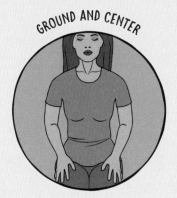

SHOULDER ROLL

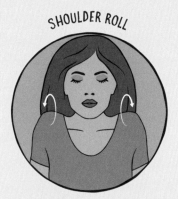

Bring your attention to the moment by sitting or standing with your feet planted firmly on the ground. Close your eyes or soften your gaze while you take a few deep breaths. Notice any sensations or sounds. Focus on feelings of tension in your body. Visualize your stress melting down through your entire body, through the soles of your feet, and out into the earth. When it feels right to do so, open your eyes. You should feel more focused, relaxed, and clear-headed.

Standing straight with your arms by your side, slowly rotate your shoulders backward, making small circles. Repeat the movement by switching the direction to forward circles.

FOREARM STRETCHES

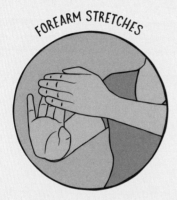

Extend your arm out with the palm and fingers facing down. Use your opposite hand to gently pull the extended hand backward toward your forearm. Hold the stretch for up to 30 seconds, then change arms and repeat.

WRIST CIRCLES

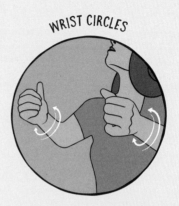

Extend both arms out and make a loose fist with each hand. Rotate your wrists ten times in slow, counterclockwise circles. Repeat in the opposite direction to make ten clockwise circles.

THUMB AND FINGER STRETCH

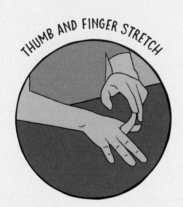

Place your hand with the palm facing down on a flat surface. One at a time, gently stretch each finger and thumb backward toward your wrist. Try not to force them farther than feels comfortable. Change hands and repeat.

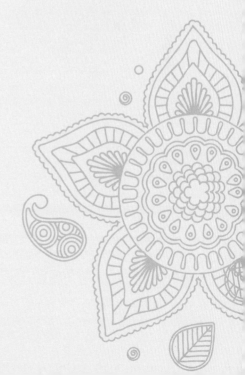

PROPS, SUPPORTS, AND BRACING

Ayurvedic head massage requires very little equipment, and is typically done best in a sturdy, upright chair, without arms. For some of the techniques described in the rituals you will need to ensure your receiver has extra support, using the techniques described here.

STRADDLE CHAIR

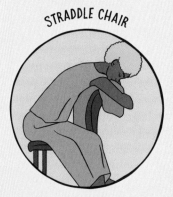

The receiver will usually sit in the chair facing out, but may find it more comfortable to sit facing the back of the chair instead. Place a large cushion between them and the chair back, covered with a towel for protection if you are using hair oil.

ROLLED TOWEL

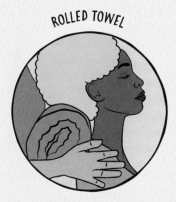

Create a comfortable place for the receiver's head to rest during compressions, shampooing, and frictions by using a rolled-up towel. Place the rolled towel on your chest or belly and encourage the receiver to lean back onto it, so they don't strain their neck muscles during the massage.

BRACING: FOREHEAD

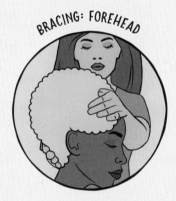

Use the forehead bracing technique to give the receiver support while applying strong strokes to the back of the neck. Stand to the receiver's left shoulder and cup their forehead in your left hand. Tilt their head forward slightly to rest in the palm of your hand. If you're left-handed, stand to your partner's right shoulder and use your right hand for support while you work with your left.

BRACING: NECK

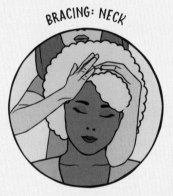

You can use this support technique while doing frictions and shampooing. Stand behind the receiver. Bend your left arm at the elbow and place your upper arm on the receiver's left shoulder. Lightly lean their head into the palm of your left hand to offer support while working on the right side. Switch the bracing technique to the receiver's right shoulder and head, using your right arm and hand, when working on the left side.

MASSAGE MOVEMENTS

With an Ayurvedic head massage we repeatedly use particular types of movement, known as massage strokes.

EFFLEURAGE

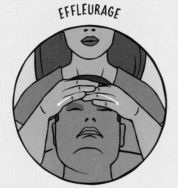

OIL APPLICATION, STROKING, HAND SWEEPING

This movement is slow, light, and rhythmic. The strokes are long and gliding, using the palms, fingers, knuckles, and forearms.

Effleurage decreases the sympathetic nervous system response, reducing muscle tension and pain.

Use effleurage to introduce your touch, apply oil, and explore the terrain before moving on to more in-depth massage techniques, and to end your massage.

PETRISSAGE

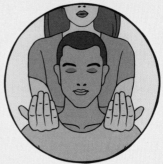

SHAMPOOING, RUFFLING, SQUEEZING, LIFTING, PINCHING, PUSHING, PULLING, ROLLING, IRONING

Petrissage means to knead. The movement uses more substantial pressure than effleurage, and involves picking up tissue. It uses the palms, fingertips, thumbs, and forearms.

FRICTIONS

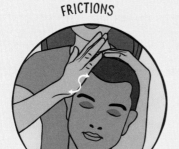

WINDSHIELD WIPER, HAIRLINE ZIGZAGS, TUGGING, SHEARING

Friction requires heavy pressure and focuses on moving the skin over the bones.

RUBS

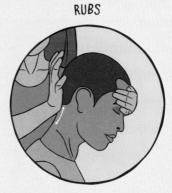

BASE OF THE SKULL RUB

A rub is a superficial movement that concentrates on rubbing over the surface of the skin.

TAPOTEMENT

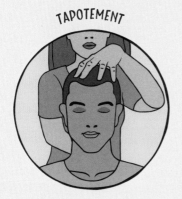

TABLA TAPPING, CHAMPI

Tapotement means to drum, strike, and tap tissues. This technique increases local circulation, wakes up muscles, and relieves general fatigue.

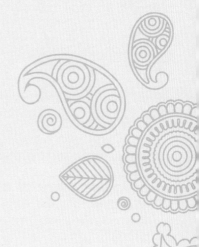

PLANTS HAVE ENOUGH SPIRIT TO
TRANSFORM OUR LIMITED VISION.

Rosemary Gladstar

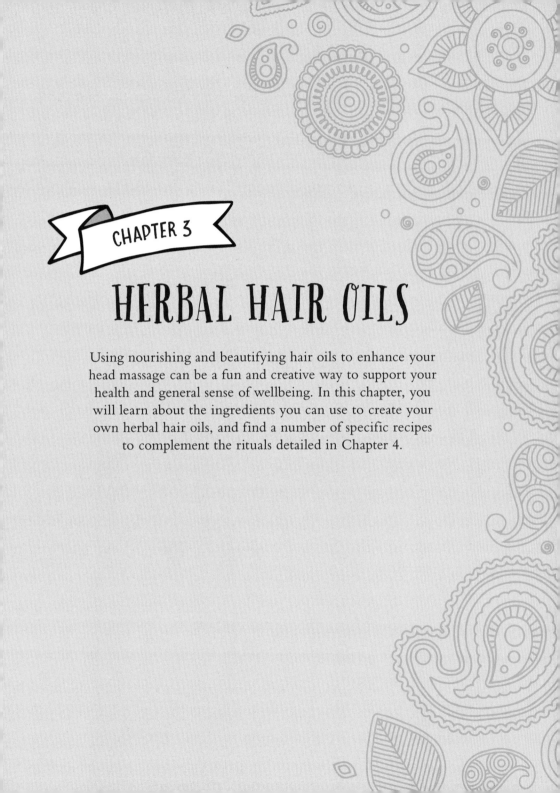

CHAPTER 3

HERBAL HAIR OILS

Using nourishing and beautifying hair oils to enhance your head massage can be a fun and creative way to support your health and general sense of wellbeing. In this chapter, you will learn about the ingredients you can use to create your own herbal hair oils, and find a number of specific recipes to complement the rituals detailed in Chapter 4.

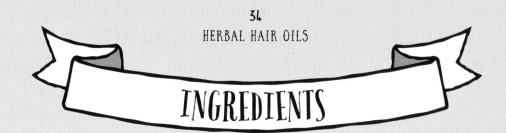

INGREDIENTS

The recipes I have created for the rituals detailed in Chapter 4 consist of essential oils suspended in a carrier oil. You can make your own mixes, following the guidelines given on page 38 regarding ratios of essential oil to carrier oil.

Use the tables on the following pages to learn a little more about the various oils and how they can support your needs.

Traditional Ayurvedic hair oils

These hair oils are ready to use.

OIL	USES
Amla (Indian gooseberry) oil	Indian gooseberry infused in coconut or sesame oil is used in Ayurveda for beauty and body care. Some formulas include brahmi, an infusion of the herb gotu kola, known for its cooling and anti-inflammatory effects. Antioxidants and nutrients strengthen the hair, making it soft and glowing.
Bhringraj oil	Bhringraj, a plant from the sunflower family, infused in sesame oil. Used to treat hair loss, premature graying, and scalp conditions.

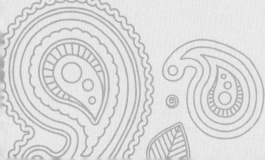

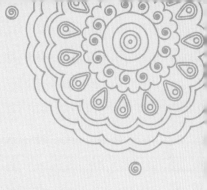

Carrier oils

A carrier oil is a nourishing plant oil used to dilute essential oils for topical use in massage and aromatherapy. These carrier oils will provide essential fatty acids, vitamins, and increase the absorption of more concentrated essential oils in your hair oil blends.

OIL	ORIGIN AND PRODUCTION	USES
Sweet almond	Almond oil, customarily found in Ayurvedic skin and hair formulas, is pressed from the almond nut and is rich in vitamin E.	Soothing and nourishing to the skin and hair.
Argan	Argan oil, pressed from the nuts of the Morrocan argan tree, is a light oil that penetrates without a greasy film.	Excellent choice for haircare because it is high in emollient and nourishing properties. Considered to be anti-aging, moisturizing, and anti-inflammatory.
Virgin coconut	Virgin coconut oil comes from the milk and the fresh meat of the coconut. It has a rich, beautiful smell of pure coconut.	Easily absorbed, softening, and moisturizing.
Jojoba	Jojoba is a liquid wax rather than an oil. It's native to the American southwest and northern Mexico, where indigenous people have used the extracts for haircare as well as for treating many health conditions.	Provides a protective barrier for the hair and skin, so is perfect for harsh climates. Antimicrobial, anti-aging, and moisturizing.
Sesame	Ayurvedic medicine makes good use of sesame oil in many formulations for health and beauty, naming it "queen of the oils."	Moisturizing, antibacterial, anti-inflammatory, and easily absorbed by the skin and hair.
Sunflower	This light oil is pressed from the blooms of the sunflower. It has a sunny disposition and is high in vitamin E.	Excellent choice for balancing and neutralizing all three doshas.

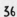
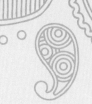

Essential oils

Essential oils are used in aromatherapy, a form of alternative medicine, as well as in wellness products to support good health. They are generally extracted from plants by distillation or other processes, such as expression, cold pressing, and solvent extraction. Essential oils in hair oil recipes can provide specific additional health benefits, as well as smelling amazing.

OIL	USES
Birch *(Betula lenulta)*	Birch oil is good for the scalp and useful for promoting hair growth. WARNING: This oil is not suitable for children and can be potentially convulsant for anyone who might be vulnerable to epileptic seizures.
Cedarwood *(Juniperus virginiana)*	Cedarwood's rejuvenating properties make it an excellent choice for oily hair and for promoting hair growth.
Chamomile (Roman) *(Anthemis nobilis)*	Chamomile's calming and anti-inflammatory properties help relieve tension, stress, and irritability.
Coriander seed *(Coriandrum sativum)*	Also known as cilantro, essential oil of coriander makes a delightful addition to shampoo or a stimulating hair oil.
Cypress *(Cupressus sempervirens)*	Cypress has been used to combat oily hair, dandruff, and is known to increase circulation in the scalp, making it excellent for haircare formulas.
Eucalyptus *(Eucalyptus globulus)*	Eucalyptus is stimulating, moisturizing, and beneficial for the health of the scalp. Its strong camphor fragrance can be emotionally supportive. WARNING: Not suitable for children under five years of age. Do not use for asthma sufferers.
Frankincense *(Boswellia thurifera)*	Frankincense helps maintain a positive mindset. It has rejuvenating, pain-relieving, and anti-inflammatory actions.
Helichrysum *(Helichrysum italicum)*	Helichrysum oil helps relieve pain and supports a healthy scalp and skin. It is emotionally uplifting and restorative.
Ho wood *(Cinnamomum camphora ct linalool)*	Ho wood is known to calm and bring about a meditative mood. It's a grounding, balancing, and introspective oil with sedative and anti-anxiety properties.

Lavender *(Lavandula angustifolia)*	Lavender neutralizes Vata energy and disperses excess Pitta and Kapha energy. It is traditionally used for relief from headaches, and to combat dry hair, hair loss, and dandruff, making it an excellent addition to any hair oil.
Lemon balm *(Melissa officinalis)*	Also known as Melissa, Lemon Balm is an excellent oil to use for stress relief and conditions of the scalp. CAUTION: Use caution for those with sensitive skin.
Orange *(Citrus sinensis)*	Orange is suitable for dry skin conditions, it also dispels anxiety, lifts sadness, and has helpful anti-inflammatory properties. ORGANIC: Non-organic citrus trees are heavily treated with pesticides that can make their way into the essential oil. Using organic orange essential oil is recommended.
Peppermint *(Mentha x piperita)*	Peppermint's cooling and moisturizing actions are excellent for calming headaches and nervous agitation. WARNING: Not suitable for children under five years of age and people with clotting disorders. Peppermint may make homeopathic remedies less effective.
Rose geranium *(Pelargonium x asperum bourbon)*	Rose geranium is very helpful for moisturizing and balancing the skin and hair.
Rose otto *(Rosa x damascena)*	Rose oil is known to calm all three dosha types. Its cooling and moisturizing actions can be helpful for nervous tension, conditions of the skin, headaches, and lifting grief.
Rosemary, ct. verbenone *(Rosemarinus officinalis ct verbenone)*	Rosemary can help prevent graying and hair loss, and reduce oil buildup. It's very stimulating to the hair and scalp and can be useful for tension headaches. CAUTION: This oil is potentially convulsant for anyone who might be vulnerable to epileptic seizures.

ESSENTIAL OIL SAFETY

- Never use an undiluted essential oil directly on the skin. If it does get on the skin, wash with soap and warm water and apply a carrier oil to the area.
- Overexposure to these potent, distilled plant oils can cause a sensitization reaction. If you experience any kind of skin reaction, discontinue use.
- Keep bottles of essential oils tightly sealed and away from the sun and other heat sources, since they can easily become oxidized and cause skin irritations. Many people like to keep their essential oils in an airtight box in the refrigerator.

RECIPES

These herbal hair oil recipes are safe for everyday use, with the essential oil content making up 2% of the mix—up to 13 drops of oil to 1 oz (30 ml) of carrier. A mix of 1% essential oil content—up to 6 drops of oil to 1 oz (30 ml) of carrier—should be used for children, the elderly, and pregnant women.

If you are allergic to any of the ingredients listed, simply take them out, or substitute them for a safer option.

USING AN OIL

Herbal hair oils may be applied before or after a head massage. In the rituals in Chapter 4, I give guidance on when you might want to use an oil, and which one to choose.

To apply an oil, pour some into your hands and massage a generous amount into the scalp and through the ends of the hair. You can leave the oil on for one to two hours, or overnight.

Shampoo and condition the hair as usual when you are ready to remove the oil. Don't forget to protect your clothes and bedding from oil stains.

Everyday hair oil

FOR THINNING HAIR
1 oz (30 ml) virgin coconut oil
3 drops coriander essential oil
3 drops birch essential oil
3 drops peppermint essential oil
3 drops Roman chamomile essential oil

Everyday hair oil

FOR DRY SCALP AND HAIR
1 oz (30 ml) unrefined sesame oil
3 drops lemon balm essential oil
3 drops rose geranium essential oil
3 drops lavender essential oil
3 drops cypress essential oil

METHOD

Pour the carrier oil into a glass bottle, ensuring there is room at the top for the essential oils.

Add the essential oils drop by drop and shake to mix.

Nourishing hair oil

1 oz (30 ml) argan oil
4 drops rosemary essential oil
2 drops cedarwood essential oil
3 drops lavender essential oil
3 drops peppermint essential oil

METHOD

Pour the carrier oil into a glass bottle, ensuring there is room at the top for the essential oils.

Add the essential oils drop by drop and shake to mix.

Reviving hair oil

1 oz (30 ml) sweet almond oil or jojoba oil
5 drops frankincense essential oil
4 drops lavender essential oil
2 drops rosemary essential oil
1 drop eucalyptus essential oil
1 drop helichrysum essential oil

METHOD

Pour the carrier oil into a glass bottle, ensuring there is room at the top for the essential oils.

Add the essential oils drop by drop and shake to mix.

Funnel the mixture into a glass bottle.

Peaceful sleep hair oil

½ oz (15 ml) virgin coconut oil
½ oz (15 ml) sesame oil
2 drops rose otto essential oil
3 drops sandalwood essential oil
1 drop ho wood essential oil

METHOD

Gently heat and blend the coconut and sesame oils in a double boiler, or use a medium-sized pan filled with 3 in. (7.5 cm) of water and a glass measuring cup for the oils.

Remove the blended oil from the heat and add the essential oils drop by drop.

Dosha balancing hair oil

1 oz (30 ml) sunflower oil
2 drops cedarwood essential oil
2 drops rose geranium essential oil
3 drops lavender essential oil
3 drops orange essential oil

METHOD

Pour the carrier oil into a glass bottle, ensuring there is room at the top for the essential oils.

Add the essential oils drop by drop and shake to mix.

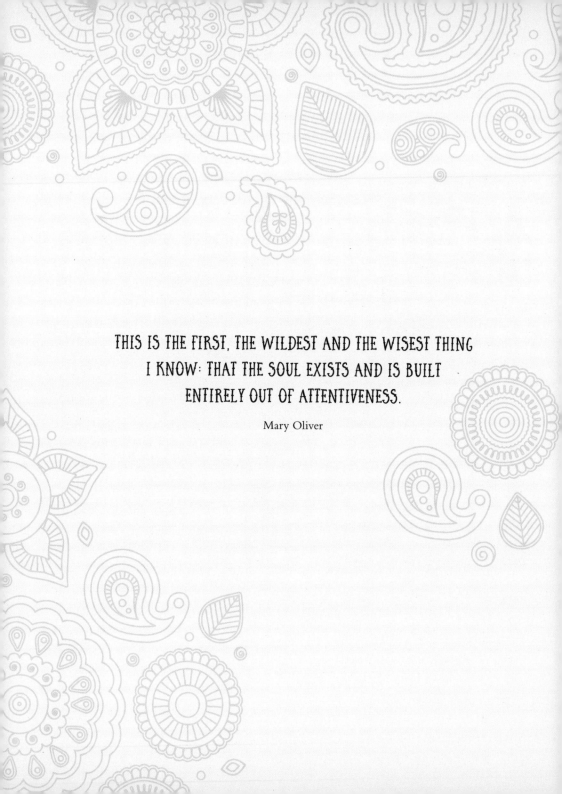

THIS IS THE FIRST, THE WILDEST AND THE WISEST THING
I KNOW: THAT THE SOUL EXISTS AND IS BUILT
ENTIRELY OUT OF ATTENTIVENESS.

Mary Oliver

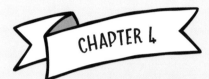

CHAPTER 4

FOCUSED INDIAN HEAD MASSAGE RITUALS

This chapter guides you through a number of massage routines that can help you to relieve symptoms of headaches and sleeplessness, lift your energy, beautify your hair and complexion, and complement individual Ayurvedic doshas. The chapter starts with the Daily Care Ritual, which teaches many of the massage techniques and marma points used in the other rituals.

Enjoy each ritual, and don't be afraid to get creative!

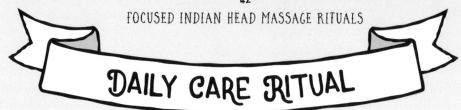

DAILY CARE RITUAL

This daily care ritual includes unique elements that form a simple Ayurvedic head massage. You'll learn invigorating movements intended to energize, as well as soothing movements that help to remove tension from your body.

The process

This ritual begins with a focus on breath and chakra balancing, moving on to stretches and massage strokes. You may finish with an application of herbal hair oil if you wish.

Chakra balancing

The breathing technique and hand positions used for the first part of the ritual are intended to balance the third-eye, throat, and crown chakras (see pages 16–17).

Herbal oil recipe

Applying a herbal oil daily might not be practical, so you may not always want to use one. However, on the days you do choose to use one, after massaging, apply the Everyday Hair Oil (see page 38).

Key massage strokes

EFFLEURAGE: PAGE 30

Sweeping; stroking

PETRISSAGE: PAGE 30

Shampooing; squeezing; lifting; pinching; rolling; pushing; pulling; ironing, compressions; ruffling

FRICTIONS: PAGE 31

Tugging; shearing; zigzags; superficial rubbing; deep friction

TAPOTEMENT: PAGE 31

Tabla tapping

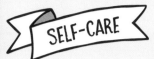
SELF-CARE

Chakra Balancing

Start this balancing sequence by closing your eyes
and noticing the natural flow of your breath.

REST AND REJUVENATE

This way of breathing stimulates your
body's autonomic nervous system to
activate its parasympathetic response,
flooding your system with hormones
that slow your heart rate and signal your
body to rest and rejuvenate.

THROAT AND THIRD EYE

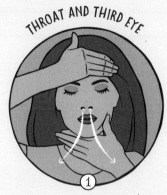

Bring the palm of one hand to hover in front
of your forehead, with the other palm in front
of your throat. Breath in and out, at your own
pace, through the nostrils only, allowing the
exhalation to resonate in the back of the
throat. Hold for five rounds of breath.

EARS

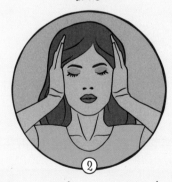

Move your palms out to cup each ear
in a relaxed position. Continue breathing
through the nostrils, and hold the position
for five rounds of breath.

EYES

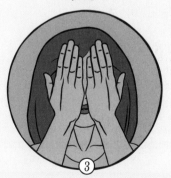

Now move the palms of your hands to lightly
cup each eye. Continue breathing through
the nostrils and hold the position for five
rounds of breath.

Stretches

Complete these stretches to prepare the muscles for the massage.

CHIN TO CHEST

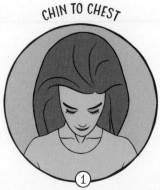

From a neutral position, exhale and bring
your chin to your chest. Hold for five to
ten seconds, breathing normally.

CHIN TO SKY

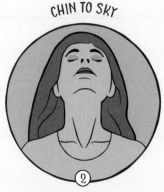

On an exhale, tilt your head back to point
your chin to the sky, and hold for five to
ten seconds, again breathing normally.

SHOULDER ROLL

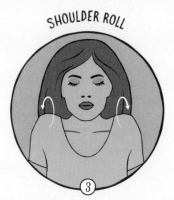

Return your head to neutral. Shrug your
shoulders up to your ears, then roll them
down and back on an exhale.

SIDE FLEXES

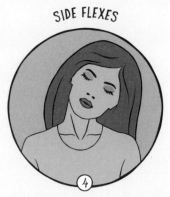

On an exhale, bring your right ear to your
right shoulder and hold for five to ten
seconds. Return to neutral on an inhale,
then repeat the stretch on the left side.

Massage Sequence

This sequence features both invigorating and soothing strokes.

SHAMPOOING

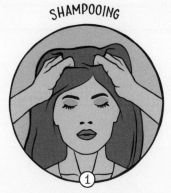

Use the fingertips and thumbs of both hands in a "shampoo-like" motion all over your head to wake up the entire scalp.

HAIR TUGGING

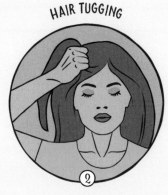

Using one hand at a time, grab fistfuls of hair at the scalp and quickly tug the hair in an upward motion at the roots. Repeat in several places all over the scalp.

TEMPLES SQUEEZE AND LIFT

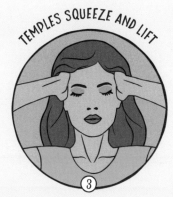

Bring the base of your palms to your temples. Simultaneously squeeze and lift toward your hairline, allowing the palms to drag the tissue in a shearing movement. Repeat three times.

EAR SQUEEZE

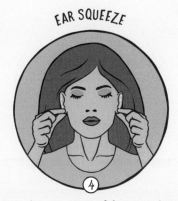

Squeeze the outer part of the ears using your forefingers and thumbs, starting at the earlobes and working up.

NECK OPENER

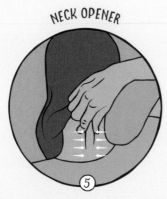

Use zigzag movements with your palm to friction all along the base of the skull. Use your right hand when working on the right side and left hand for the left side.

ZIGZAG FRICTIONS

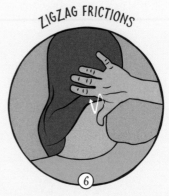

Use zigzag movements with your palm to friction all along the base of the skull. Use your right hand when working on the right side and left hand for the left side.

SHOULDER SQUEEZE

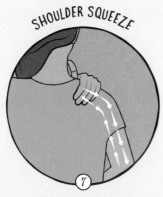

Use your left hand to gently squeeze the tissue of your right shoulder near the neck. Repeat at intervals moving along the shoulder and down the upper arm to the elbow. Work back up the arm in the same way. Make three rounds and repeat on the other side.

COVER UP

If you choose to apply a herbal hair oil after the massage, make sure you wear clothing that you don't mind getting stained or messy.

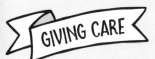

Chakra Balancing

To begin, focus, connect, and engage with the receiver's chakras.

FOCUS

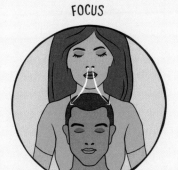

In order to focus and bring your attention to the present moment, take a deep breath and bring the palms of your hands together in front of your chest.

CONNECTION

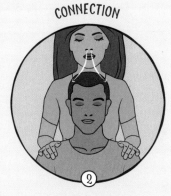

When you are ready, gently rest your palms on the receiver's shoulders. Breathe in and out through the nostrils only, allowing the exhalation to resonate in the back of your throat. Hold for three rounds of breath, breathing at your own pace.

THIRD EYE

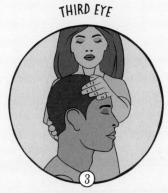

Move to stand facing the receiver's left shoulder. Place the palm of your left hand lightly on their forehead and cup your right palm at the base of their skull, just above the neck. Hold for three rounds of breath.

CROWN

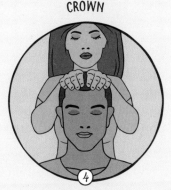

Move to stand behind the receiver and gently rest the palms of your hands on the crown of their head. Hold for three rounds of breath.

Stretches

Stretching is a great way to prepare the muscles and connective tissues for massage.

HAND PLACEMENT

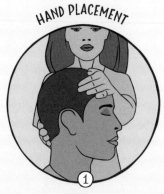

Stand facing the receiver's left shoulder. Place the palm of your left hand over the receiver's forehead and your right palm on the back of their head, just above the neck.

CHIN TO CHEST

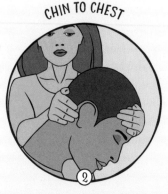

Ask the receiver to take a deep breath. On their exhale, slowly bring their chin to their chest.

CHIN TO SKY

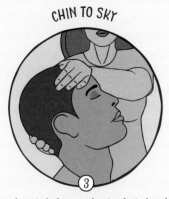

When they inhale, gently tip their head back so that their chin points to the sky. Slowly and methodically continue the Chin to Chest and Chin to Sky sequence, following the breath pattern, for a total of three rounds.

RECEIVER'S COMFORT
When you're moving someone else's neck, work slowly and mindfully, and check in with them regularly regarding their comfort.

Massage Sequence

This ritual includes many of the elements found in each of the massage rituals.

SHOULDER SWEEP

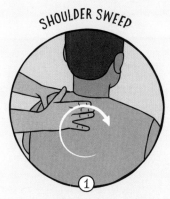

Place your left hand on the receiver's left shoulder for stability. Relax and warm up the shoulders by rubbing the upper back in large, clockwise, circular movements with the palm of your right hand. Use medium pressure and focus around the shoulder blades.

SHOULDER PUSH AND PULLS

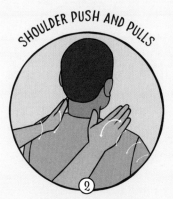

Standing behind the receiver, place the base of each palm at the top of each shoulder blade. Using medium pressure with your palms, push the muscles forward, moving up and over. Pull the muscles back by dragging your fingers toward you. Repeat at intervals along the shoulder toward the arm.

SHOULDER SQUEEZE

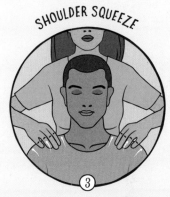

Wrap your fingers around the front and thumbs behind the shoulders. Grab the muscle on the top and squeeze with medium pressure. Hold for a few seconds. Repeat at the middle of the shoulders and again near the base of the neck. Repeat this sequence three times.

GIVER'S COMFORT

Remember to keep your own shoulders down and relaxed.

IRONING OUT I

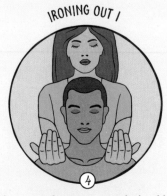

Place your forearms on each shoulder
near the base of the neck. With your
hands slightly higher than your elbows,
turn your palms to face upward.

IRONING OUT II

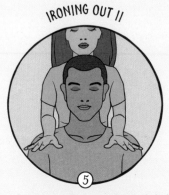

Using firm to medium pressure, slide both
forearms simultaneously across the top of the
shoulders, twisting your arms so the palms
face the ground as you come to the end of the
movement. Repeat the whole Ironing Out
sequence a total of three times.

IRONING DOWN I

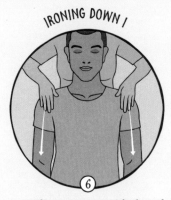

Now use medium pressure with the palms and
heels of your hands to compress the muscles
from the top of the arms down to the elbows.

IRONING DOWN II

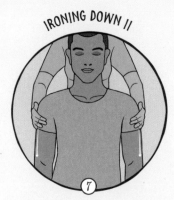

Use the same technique to compress
down the sides of the arms.

IRONING DOWN ///

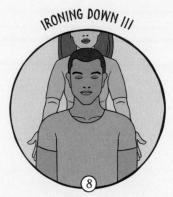

8

Finally, using light pressure, iron down the back of the arms. Repeat the whole Ironing Down sequence three times.

PALM ROLL

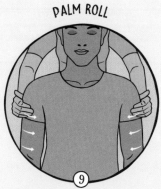

9

Place your hands on the receiver's upper arms, with your fingers in front and the base of your palms behind. With medium pressure, roll the palms forward over the muscles to meet your fingertips, being careful not to pinch the skin. Repeat in the middle of the upper arm, and then again just above the elbow. Repeat the whole process three times.

NECK OPENER

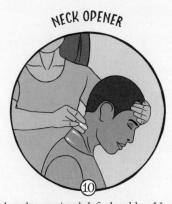

10

Stand at the receiver's left shoulder. Use your left hand to cup their forehead for support. Tilt the head forward into your hand slightly. Bring your right hand to the top of the neck, grab the flesh there and pull it back. Grab at the middle of the neck and pull back again, then repeat at the base of the neck. Repeat the entire sequence a total of three times.

RECEIVER'S SUPPORT

Use the forehead bracing technique to give the receiver support while applying strong strokes to the back of the neck. If you're left-handed, stand to the receiver's right shoulder and use your right hand for support while you work with your left.

NECK PUSHES AND PULLS I

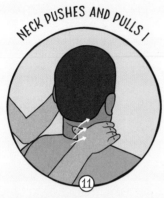

With their forehead still in your left palm, place your right thumb at the top of the receiver's neck, to the left of the spine. Push the thumb forward diagonally across the side of the neck. Repeat this movement in the middle and at the base of the neck.

NECK PUSHES AND PULLS II

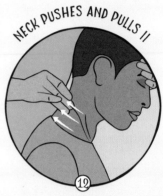

Position two or three fingers close to the spine with your thumb anchored on the other side. Pull your fingers back toward your thumb. Repeat at the middle and top of the neck. Repeat the Pushes and Pulls sequence for a total of three passes, then change hands and repeat on the other side of the neck.

FINGERTIP FRICTION

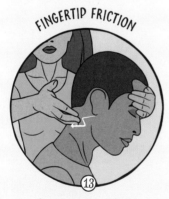

Use your fingertips to apply friction in a zigzag motion along the base of the skull to relax the muscles underneath the occipital bone. Start behind the ear and move toward the midline, avoiding the spine. Switch hands and repeat on the other side.

HEEL RUB

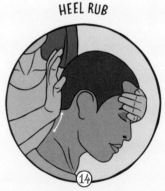

With one hand still on the receiver's forehead, rub the base of the skull lightly and briskly with the heel and palm of the other hand in an up-and-down movement.

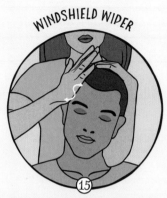

WINDSHIELD WIPER

15

Stand behind the receiver and support one
side of their head using the bracing technique.
Use the heel of the other hand to lightly rub
over one side of the head, moving your hand
from side to side, like a windshield wiper.

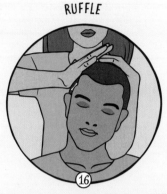

RUFFLE

16

Next, use your whole hand to ruffle
the top of the receiver's head. Repeat
Steps 15–16 on the other side of the head,
then continue with two more rounds,
alternating between each side.

BRACING

The neck bracing technique will provide
support for the receiver during frictions.
Stand behind the receiver and bend one
arm at the elbow. Place the bent arm on
the receiver's shoulder and lightly lean
their head into the palm of your hand
to offer support while working on the
opposite side of the head.

WHOLE HAND FRICTION I

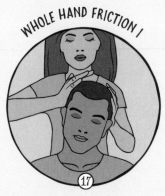

Standing behind the receiver, support one side of their head and place your other hand above the opposite ear. Apply firm pressure to move the scalp up and down. Repeat on the other side.

WHOLE HAND FRICTION II

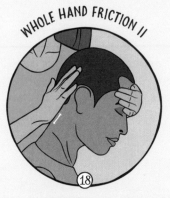

Stand to one side of the receiver with one hand at the base of their skull. Apply firm pressure to move the scalp up and down. Repeat on the other side.

WHOLE HAND FRICTION III

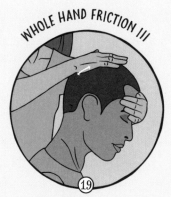

Repeat the friction action on the top of the head.

RUFFLING

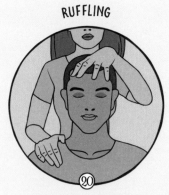

With one hand on the receiver's shoulder, use the fingers of the other hand to ruffle their hair, keeping light contact with the scalp. Toss long hair at the nape of the neck. Keep your touch light.

TABLA TAPPING

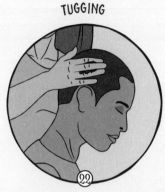

Use your fingertips to gently tap all over the scalp: imagine that you're playing a piano.

TUGGING

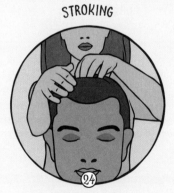

Slide one hand forward through the hair, keeping your fingers and palms in contact with the scalp. Bring your fingers together, gripping the hair at the base. Move your hand from side to side, moving the scalp. Do this in several places, then repeat with the other hand on the other side of the head.

SHAMPOOING

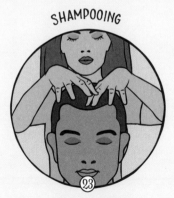

Use medium pressure with the fingertips and thumbs of both hands in a "shampoo-like" motion all over the scalp.

STROKING

Bring one hand flat over the top of the head with fingers pointing toward the hairline. Slowly rake through the hair, following with the other hand in a wave-like motion. Continue to the sides of the head, stopping at the ears. Repeat five to seven times.

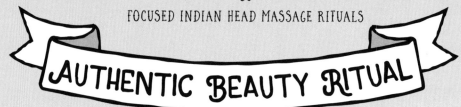

AUTHENTIC BEAUTY RITUAL

The authentic beauty ritual enhances radiance and natural beauty. This ritual stimulates marma energy points and uses special massage techniques to address excess fluid in the face, release tension in the jaw and brow lines, and support healthy circulation through the scalp. You'll encourage glossy hair, a healthy scalp, and a clearer, more vibrant complexion, all while relaxing your mind, body, and spirit.

The process

This ritual begins with marma energy work, followed by massage techniques and an application of herbal hair oil if you wish.

Marma points

You will be stimulating the Arshak, Manya, Brahma Randra, and Murdhi marma points (see pages 18–21). Stimulating the Arshak point supports lymphatic drainage for a clear complexion; the Manya improves circulation; the Brahma Randra supports hormonal balance; and Murdhi brings feelings of joy that can radiate in your outward appearance.

Herbal oil recipe

After massaging you can apply the Nourishing Hair Oil (see page 39). Let the oil sit for at least one hour, or overnight. You can also dot your fingertips with oil when stimulating the marma points.

Key massage strokes

EFFLEURAGE: PAGE 30

Circular; sweeping; stroking

PETRISSAGE: PAGE 30

Squeezing; pinching; ruffling; pulling; shampooing

FRICTIONS: PAGE 31

Zigzags; tugging; scrubbing

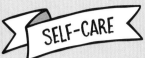

Marma Sequence

Use your middle and ring fingers in slow, clockwise circles—seven is a good
number; however, if you are new to Ayurvedic head massage then three circles may
be preferable. You can use a herbal oil for this sequence if you wish. Refer to pages
18–21 for extra guidance with locating the points.

ARSHAK

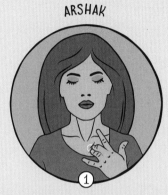

The Arshak points are located on each side of
your body, just above the clavicle. Stimulate
one side with seven slow, clockwise circles
and repeat on the other side.

MANYA

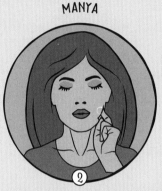

Locate the Manya point, four finger-widths
below the earlobe. Stimulate one side with
seven slow, clockwise circles and repeat on
the other side.

BRAHMA RANDRA

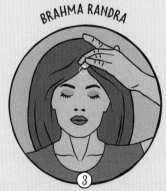

The Brahma Randra point is located at the
center of the scalp just above the hairline.
Massage this point using light pressure and
seven slow, clockwise circles.

MURDHI

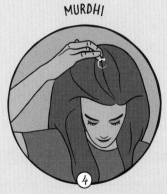

Locate the Murdhi marma point. Massage
using light pressure, moving your fingers in
slow, clockwise circles seven times.

Massage Sequence

Use this sequence to enhance local circulation to the head and hair, encourage a
clear complexion, and bring a sense of balance and joy.

NECK OPENER

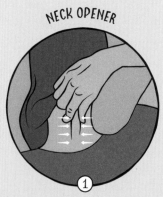

Starting at the top and moving down, squeeze
the back of the neck with the right hand,
focusing on areas of tension. Repeat with
the left hand.

NECK PUMPS

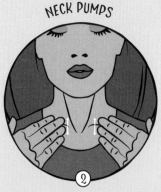

Place the fingertips of each hand above each
collarbone and use gentle up and down
pumping motions to help drain lymphatic
fluid away from the neck and face. Do this
motion 50 times.

JAWLINE SWEEP

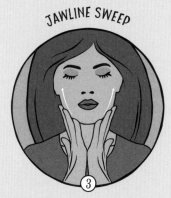

Bring your hands together in front of your
chin, with fingers slightly open. Use slow,
sweeping motions to follow the jawline up
toward the ears. Repeat three times.

TEMPLE CIRCLES

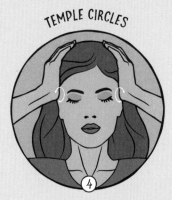

Squeeze the temples with the base of the
palms while making slow, large, circular
movements. Make three circles in a clockwise
direction and three counterclockwise.

FOREHEAD GLIDES

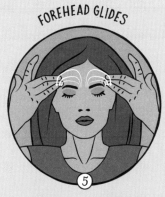

Place the middle and ring fingers of each hand between the eyebrows. Using gentle pressure, glide the fingers straight up and out to follow your hairline. Repeat the action midway between the hairline and eyebrow, and once more right above the eyebrows. Complete the sequence three times in total.

BROW BONE PINCH

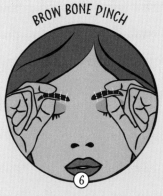

Beginning close to the nose, lightly pinch the eyebrows all along the brow bone between thumbs and forefingers. Work out to the ends of the eyebrows. Complete three passes.

ZIGZAGS

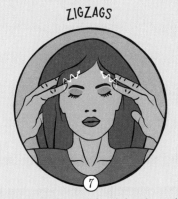

With the fingertips of each hand, quickly scrub the entire hairline back and forth in a zigzag pattern. Don't forget the back of the head.

RUFFLING

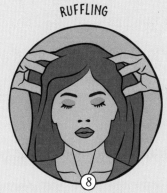

Using the fingers of both hands, briskly ruffle your hair keeping light contact with the scalp. Toss and flick long hair at the nape of the neck. Keep your touch light.

HAIR TUGGING

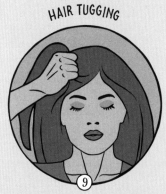

Using one hand at a time, grab fistfuls of hair at the scalp and quickly tug the hair in an upward motion at the roots. Repeat in several places all over the scalp.

SHAMPOOING

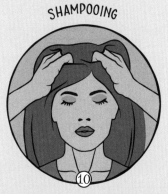

Use medium pressure with the fingertips and thumbs of both hands in a "shampoo-like" motion all over the scalp.

PILLOW PROTECTION

If you plan to keep a herbal hair oil on overnight, make sure you protect your pillow with a towel, or use an old pillowcase that you don't mind getting stained or messy.

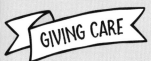

Marma Sequence

Use your middle and ring fingers in slow, clockwise circles—if you are new to head massage you may prefer to make three, not seven, circles. You can use a herbal oil if you wish. Refer to pages 18–21 for guidance with locating the points.

ARSHAK

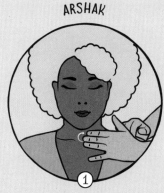

The Arshak points are located on each side of your body, just above the clavicle. Stimulate one side with seven slow, clockwise circles and repeat on the other side.

MANYA

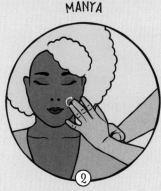

Locate the Manya point, four finger-widths below the earlobe. Stimulate one side with seven slow, clockwise circles and repeat on the other side.

BRAHMA RANDRA

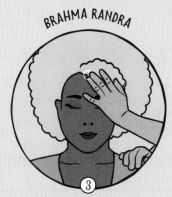

The Brahma Randra point is located at the center of the scalp just above the hairline. Massage this point using light pressure and seven slow, clockwise circles.

MURDHI

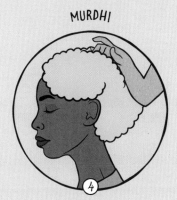

Standing behind the receiver, locate the Murdhi point and make seven slow, clockwise circles.

Massage Sequence

Use this sequence to support family and friends with overall beauty, good health, and wellness.

SHOULDER SQUEEZE

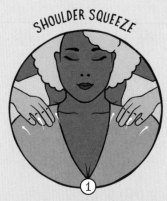

Place your hands on the outside edge of the shoulders with your fingers in front and thumbs behind. Squeeze the muscle on top of the shoulders with medium pressure. Hold for a few seconds, then release. Repeat at the middle of the shoulders, and again near the base of the neck. Make a total of three passes.

NECK OPENER

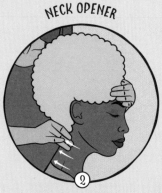

Stand at the receiver's left shoulder. Use your left hand to cup their forehead for support. Tilt the head forward into your hand slightly. Bring your right hand to the top of the neck, grab the flesh there and pull it back. Grab at the middle of the neck and pull back again, then repeat at the base of the neck. Repeat the entire sequence a total of three times.

STABILIZE

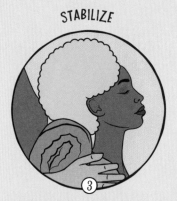

Stand behind the receiver and use a rolled towel to stabilize their head for the next sequence.

TOWEL STABILIZING

The rolled-towel method of support is useful when applying compressions, shampooing, and frictions. Place a rolled towel on your chest or belly and ask the receiver to lean back onto it, so they don't strain their neck muscles during the massage.

JAWLINE SWEEP

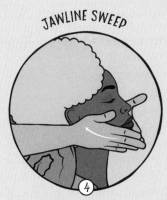

(4)

Bring your fingertips together creating a "V" shape in line with the receiver's chin. Using light pressure, sweep up the jawline. Make three sweeps in total.

LIP SWEEP

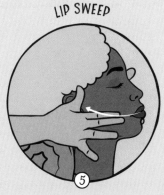

(5)

Using the middle and ring fingers of each hand, lightly sweep from the center of the lips out toward the ears. Repeat to make three sweeps in total.

CHEEKBONE SWEEP

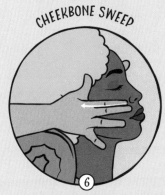

(6)

Place the middle and ring fingers of each hand on either side of the nose and sweep under the cheekbones out toward the ears. Make three sweeps in total.

FOREHEAD SWEEP

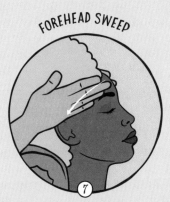

(7)

Bring the fingers of each hand together and place them on the forehead. Broadly sweep from the center out toward the temples. Repeat twice more.

TEMPLE CIRCLES

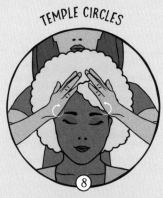

(8)

Bring the base of your palms to the receiver's temples. Using medium pressure, squeeze and lift toward the hairline. Make three large circles over the temples.

BRACING

The neck bracing technique will provide support for the receiver during frictions. Stand behind the receiver and bend one arm at the elbow. Place the bent arm on the receiver's shoulder and lightly lean their head into the palm of your hand to offer support while working on the opposite side of the head.

HAIRLINE ZIGZAGS

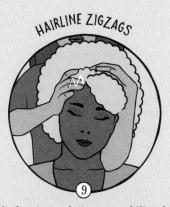

(9)

Use the bracing technique to stabilize the left side of the receiver's neck. Make short and quick zigzag movements with the fingertips of your right hand back and forth along the hairline on the right side. Complete three passes in total.

SCALP ZIGZAGS

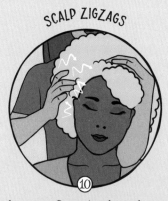

(10)

Now place your fingertips above the receiver's ear on the right side. Apply firm pressure to briskly rub across the entire right side of the scalp in a zigzag movement three times. Switch sides and repeat the whole Hairline and Scalp Zigzag sequence on the left side.

RUFFLING

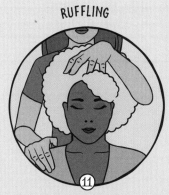

With one hand on the receiver's shoulder, use the fingers of the other hand to ruffle their hair, keeping light contact with the scalp. Toss long hair at the nape of the neck. Keep your touch light.

SHAMPOOING

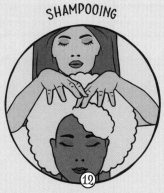

Use medium pressure with the fingertips and thumbs of both hands in a "shampoo-like" motion all over the scalp.

STROKING

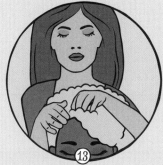

Standing behind the receiver, bring one hand flat over the top of the head with your fingers pointing toward the beginning of the hairline, and slowly rake through the hair. Follow with the other hand in a wave-like pattern.

PILLOW PROTECTION

If the receiver would like to keep a herbal hair oil on overnight, remind them to protect their pillow with a towel, or use an old pillowcase that they don't mind getting stained or messy.

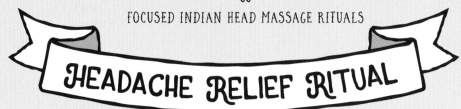

HEADACHE RELIEF RITUAL

Tension headaches are usually caused by fatigue, the daily stresses of hectic lifestyles, and chronic worry. As a result, muscles often become tight and restricted in the shoulders, neck, jaw, face, and scalp. This targeted ritual was created to naturally soothe tension headaches. Using it regularly can help you adapt to the chaos of daily life and reduce the frequency of tension headaches.

The process

This ritual begins with stretches, followed by marma energy work. Massage techniques address stress-related tension in the neck, shoulders, head, and face.

Marma points

You will be stimulating the Kirkatika, Bhruh, and Murdhi points, and when giving care you can also stimulate the Shankha point (see pages 18–21). Massaging the Kirkatika point helps to relieve pain in the back of the head; Bhruh may help with some migraine symptoms; and stimulating Murdhi helps to relieve neck and back tension while relaxing the entire body.

Herbal oil recipe

If you want to use an oil for the massage, choose the Reviving Hair Oil (see page 39). You can also use a little oil on your fingers when stimulating the marma points.

Key massage strokes

EFFLEURAGE: PAGE 30
Circular; sweeping

PETRISSAGE: PAGE 30
Squeezing; lifting; shampooing

FRICTIONS: PAGE 31
Pulling; shearing; zigzags

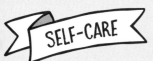

Stretches

Use both hands to pin the pectoral muscle on the right side, then follow the stretch steps. Once the whole sequence is complete, swap the hand position and repeat on the other side.

EAR TO SHOULDER

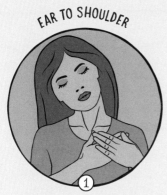

With your hands pinned to the right side, take your left ear toward your left shoulder and hold for five seconds.

CHIN TO SHOULDER

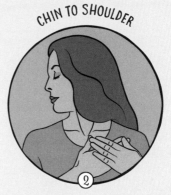

Gently change position so your chin now faces your left shoulder. Hold for five seconds.

CHIN TO THE SKY

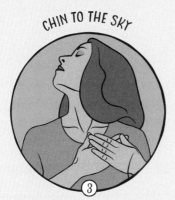

Gently move your chin to face up, in line with your shoulder, and hold for five seconds. Repeat the entire sequence on the right side.

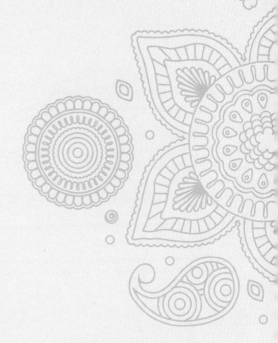

Marma Sequence

Use your middle and ring fingers in slow, clockwise circles—if you are new to Ayurvedic head massage you can make three, not seven, circles. You can use a herbal oil if you wish. Refer to pages 18–21 for guidance with locating the points.

KIRKATIKA

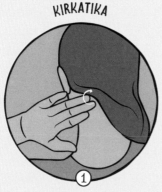

Place the middle and ring fingers of your left hand at the base of the skull where it meets the neck on the left side. Make seven slow, clockwise circles. Repeat on the right side using your right hand.

BHRUH

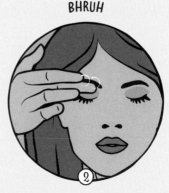

Use your left middle finger to locate the inner end of your left eyebrow, close to the bridge of the nose. Using slow, clockwise circles, work along the brow bone toward the outer edge of the eyebrow. Search for tiny bumps or indentations. Repeat on the other side.

SHANKHA

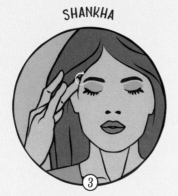

Use your left ring and middle fingers to locate the hollow of your left temple. Make seven slow, clockwise circles. Repeat on the right temple using your other hand.

Massage Sequence

These massage techniques address stress-related tension in the neck, shoulders, head, and face.

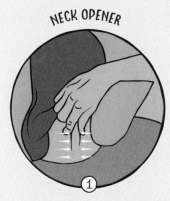

NECK OPENER

Squeeze the back of the neck with the right hand in intervals, starting from the top of the neck and moving down. Repeat with the left hand.

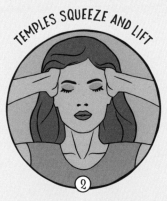

TEMPLES SQUEEZE AND LIFT

Bring the base of your palms to your temples. Simultaneously squeeze and lift toward the hairline, allowing the palms to drag the tissue in a shearing movement. Repeat three times.

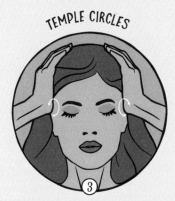

TEMPLE CIRCLES

Now use the base of the palms to make slow, clockwise circles at the temples. Make three circles in total.

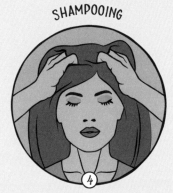

SHAMPOOING

Use medium pressure with the fingertips and thumbs of both hands in a "shampoo-like" motion all over the scalp.

EYE CIRCLES

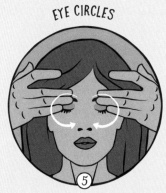

Use the pads of the ring and middle fingers to lightly sweep from the center of the eyebrow along the brow bone and around the eye to the nose. Complete three passes in total.

JAWLINE SWEEP

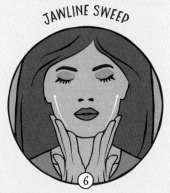

Bring your hands together in front of your chin. Point your fingers toward your chin and slightly open them. Use slow, sweeping motions to follow the jawline up toward the ears. Repeat three times.

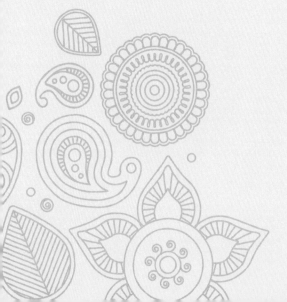

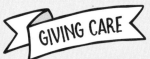

Stretches

The tissues in the upper back and neck can become tense and stuck, causing frequent tension headaches. Incorporating movement through stretches before the massage can be a valuable tool to warm up the tissues and inform you as to where to focus the massage.

HAND PLACEMENT

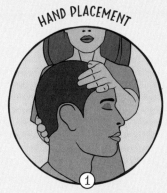

Stand facing the receiver's left shoulder. Place the palm of your left hand over the receiver's forehead and your right palm on the back of their head, just above the neck.

CHIN TO CHEST

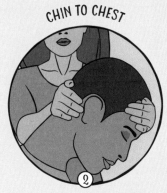

Ask the receiver to take a deep breath. On their exhale, slowly bring their chin to their chest.

CHIN TO SKY

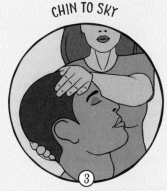

When they inhale, gently tip their head back so that their chin points to the sky. Slowly and methodically continue the Chin to Chest and Chin to Sky sequence, following the breath pattern, for a total of three rounds.

RECEIVER'S COMFORT

When moving someone else's neck, work slowly and mindfully, and check in with them regularly regarding their comfort.

Marma Sequence

Use your middle and ring fingers in slow, clockwise circles—if you are new to head massage you may prefer to make three, not seven, circles. You can use a herbal oil if you wish. Refer to pages 18–21 for guidance with locating the points.

KIRKATIKA

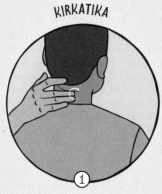

1

Locate the Kirkatika point at the base of the skull where it meets the neck on the right side. Make seven slow, clockwise circles. Repeat on the left side.

MURDHI

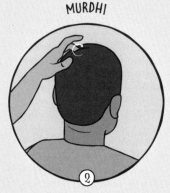

2

Standing behind the receiver, locate the Murdhi point with your middle and ring fingers and make seven slow, clockwise circles.

SHANKHA

3

Locate the Shankha point in the hollows of the temples. Stimulate one side with seven slow, clockwise circles, then repeat on the other side.

BHRUH

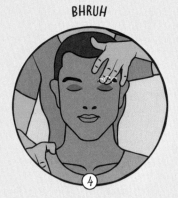

4

Standing behind the receiver, place the ring and middle fingers at the end of one eyebrow, close to the nose. Using slow, clockwise circles, work along the brow bone, searching for tiny bumps or indentations. Switch hands to repeat on the other side.

Massage Sequence

Combined with the stretching of tight muscles and stimulating marma points for increased circulation, this tension-taming massage sequence will give relief from even the most intense headache.

SHOULDER SQUEEZE

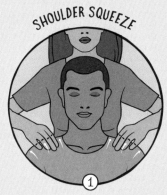

NECK OPENER

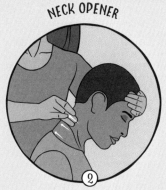

Place your hands on the outside edge of the shoulders with your fingers in front and thumbs behind. Squeeze the muscle on top of the shoulders with medium pressure. Hold for a few seconds, then release. Repeat at the middle of the shoulders, and again near the base of the neck. Make a total of three passes.

Stand at the receiver's left shoulder. Use your left hand to cup their forehead for support. Tilt the head forward into your hand slightly. Bring your right hand to the top of the neck, grab the flesh there and pull it back. Grab at the middle of the neck and pull back again, then repeat at the base of the neck. Repeat the entire sequence a total of three times.

RECEIVER'S SUPPORT

Use the forehead bracing technique to give the receiver support while applying strong strokes to the back of the neck. If you're left-handed, stand to the receiver's right shoulder and use your right hand for support while you work with your left.

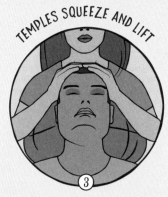

TEMPLES SQUEEZE AND LIFT

③

Stand behind the receiver and use a rolled towel to stabilize their head. Bring the base of your palms to their temples and gently squeeze and lift toward the hairline.

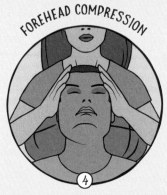

FOREHEAD COMPRESSION

④

Bring the fingers of each hand together and place them on the forehead. Gently press and shear toward the ears.

TOWEL STABILIZING

The rolled-towel method of support is useful when applying compressions and frictions. Place a rolled towel on your chest or belly and ask the receiver to lean back onto it, so they don't strain their neck muscles during the massage.

SHAMPOOING

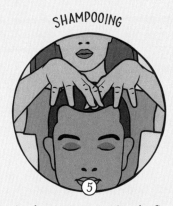

(5)

Make circular movements using the fingertips and thumbs of both hands in a "shampoo-like" motion. Repeat all over the scalp, starting with slow movements, then try slightly quicker. Pay special attention to the temporalis muscles on each side of the head.

VERTICAL ZIGZAGS I

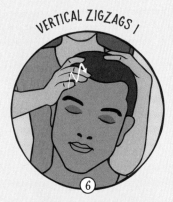

(6)

Make short, quick zigzag movements with the fingertips of your right hand on the right side of the receiver's scalp. Working upward each time, start along the hairline to the temples.

VERTICAL ZIGZAGS II

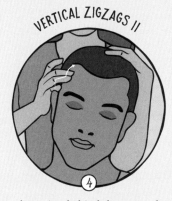

(4)

Repeat the action behind the ear, and again at the back of the head. Repeat with the left hand for the left side of the scalp.

BRACING

The neck bracing technique provides support for the receiver during frictions. Stand behind the receiver and bend one arm at the elbow. Place the bent arm on the receiver's shoulder and lightly lean their head into the palm of your hand to offer support while working on the opposite side of the head.

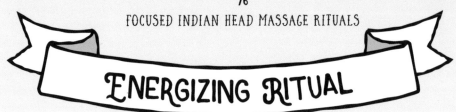

ENERGIZING RITUAL

Midday is the perfect time to take a break for a revitalizing Ayurvedic head massage. This energizing ritual is a healthy pick-me-up for those days when you have low energy but your to-do list is looming. It's easy to get stuck on a task, but planning a break from your hectic day can actually help you to be more productive.

The process

This ritual begins with neck stretches, followed by marma energy work to support vitality, focus, and memory. The brisk massage that follows will leave the receiver feeling more awake and ready to take on any task.

Marma points

You will be stimulating the Ushta, Nasa, Gandu, Avarta, Shankha, and Ajna marma points (see pages 18–21). The Ushta point promotes awareness and concentration; the Nasa point helps you to feel clear-headed; stimulating the Gandu point can rejuvenate tired eyes; Avarta helps with alertness; Shankha for focus; and Ajna awakens wisdom.

Herbal oil recipe

If you want to use an oil for the massage, choose the Reviving Hair Oil (see page 39). You can also use a little oil on your fingers when stimulating the marma points.

Key massage strokes

EFFLEURAGE: PAGE 30
Circular; sweeping

PETRISSAGE: PAGE 30
Ruffling; squeezing

FRICTIONS: PAGE 31
Zigzags; plucking; whole hand friction; pulling; champi

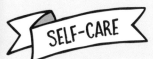

SELF-CARE

Stretches

For this stretching sequence, imagine your chin drawing an infinity symbol
(figure eight on its side) in the air. Start with side flexes (see page 44), then
repeat the Infinity sequence three times in total, moving slowly and noticing
where you're holding tension in your neck.

INFINITY I

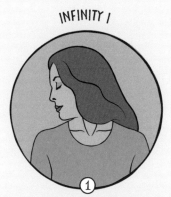

Loosen the neck a little with side flexes (see
page 44). Next, as you exhale, bring your chin
to your left shoulder. Hold for three breaths.

INFINITY II

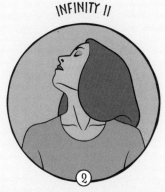

Lift your chin up and slightly tilt your head
back, so that you are looking at the ceiling.

INFINITY III

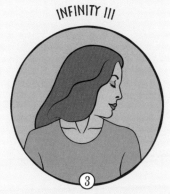

In the air, draw half of an infinity sign with
your chin, bringing your right ear to your
right shoulder.

INFINITY IV

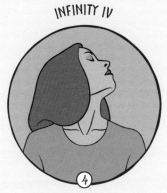

Repeat the Infinity sequence in the other
direction. After three rounds, bring your head
back to a neutral position.

Marma Sequence

Use your middle and ring fingers in slow, clockwise circles—seven is a good number; however, if you are new to Ayurvedic head massage then three circles may be preferable. You can use a herbal oil for this sequence if you wish. Refer to pages 18–21 for guidance with locating the points.

USHTA

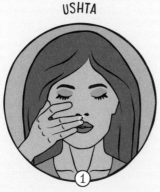

Use your middle and ring fingers to locate the Ushta point in the center of the upper lip. Massage using seven slow, clockwise circles.

NASA

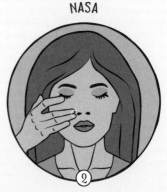

The Nasa point is found where the flared parts of the nostrils join the face on either side of the nose. Stimulate one side with seven slow, clockwise circles, then repeat on the other side of the nose.

GANDU

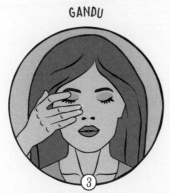

Locate the Gandu point halfway up the side of the nose. Stimulate one side with seven slow, clockwise circles, then repeat on the other side of the nose.

AVARTA

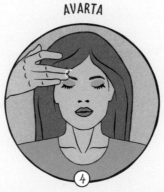

The Avarta point is found on the forehead, in the middle of each eyebrow. Massage using seven slow, clockwise circles.

SHANKHA

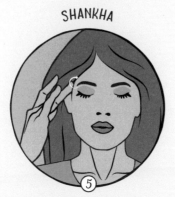

Use your left ring and middle fingers to locate the hollow of your left temple. Make seven slow, clockwise circles. Repeat on the other temple using your right hand.

AJNA

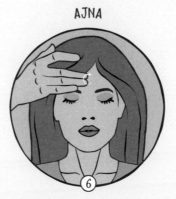

This point is known as the third-eye point, and is found in the center of the forehead. Use the middle and ring fingers to make seven slow, clockwise circles.

Massage Sequence

Make your movements brisk for this massage, to encourage the energizing effect.

EYE SOOTHER

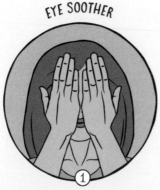

Cup your hands and place them over your eyes. Stay in this position for roughly one minute, allowing the muscles of your eyes to relax and to alleviate eye strain.

RUFFLING

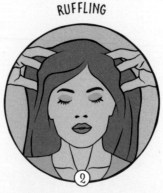

Using the fingers of both hands, briskly ruffle your hair keeping light contact with the scalp. Toss and flick long hair at the nape of the neck. Keep your touch light.

VERTICAL ZIGZAGS

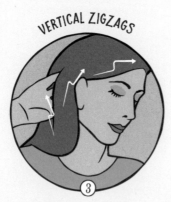

Make short and quick zigzag movements with the fingertips of one hand on the same side of your scalp. Working upward each time, start along your hairline to the temples, repeat the action behind the ear, and again at the back of the head. Repeat with the other hand for the other side of the scalp.

PLUCKING

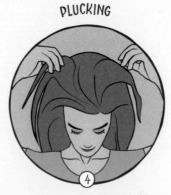

With your fingers long, land softly on the head and spring off quickly, bringing your fingers and thumbs together. Repeat this movement in different places until you've covered your entire scalp.

EAR SQUEEZE

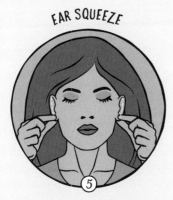

Squeeze the outer part of the ears using your forefingers and thumbs, starting at the earlobes and working up.

EAR PULL

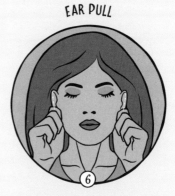

Using light pressure, slowly pull the ears up and down, starting at the earlobes and working up.

NECK OPENER

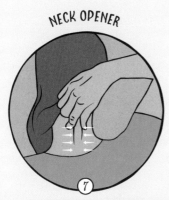

Squeeze the back of the neck with the right hand at intervals, starting from the top of the neck and moving down. Repeat with the left hand.

SHOULDER SQUEEZE

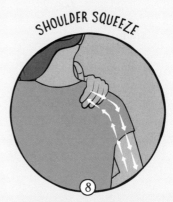

Use your left hand to gently squeeze the tissue of your right shoulder near the neck. Repeat at intervals moving along the shoulder and down the upper arm to the elbow. Work back up the arm in the same way. Make three rounds and repeat on the other side.

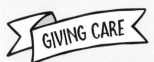

Marma Sequence

Ask the receiver to complete the stretches detailed on page 77, then use the middle and ring fingers in slow, clockwise circles—if you are new to Ayurvedic head massage you may prefer to make three, not seven, circles. You can use a herbal oil if you wish. Refer to pages 18–21 for guidance with locating the points.

AVARTA

SHANKHA

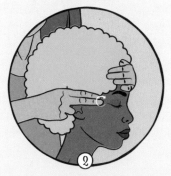

After stretching (see page 77), locate the Avarta point on the forehead, directly in the middle of each eyebrow. Massage using seven slow, clockwise circles.

Locate the Shankha point in the hollows of the temples. Stimulate one side with seven slow, clockwise circles, then repeat on the other side.

AJNA

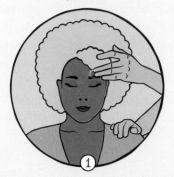

Ajna is known as the third eye-point, and is located in the center of the forehead. Use the middle and ring fingers to make seven slow, clockwise circles.

Massage Sequence

Keep your massage movements brisk and lively to avoid a sedating effect.
Remember to also be responsive to the receiver's preferences regarding
movement and pressure.

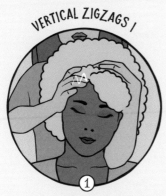

VERTICAL ZIGZAGS I

Make short, quick zigzag movements with the
fingertips of your right hand on the right side
of the receiver's scalp. Working upward each
time, start along the hairline to the temples.

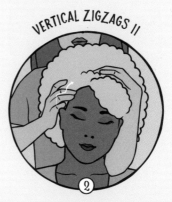

VERTICAL ZIGZAGS II

Repeat the action behind the ear, and again at
the back of the head. Repeat with the left
hand for the left side of the scalp.

BRACING

The neck bracing technique will provide
support for the receiver during frictions.
Stand behind the receiver and bend one
arm at the elbow. Place the bent arm on
the receiver's shoulder and lightly lean
their head into the palm of your hand to
offer support while working on the
opposite side of the head.

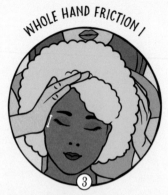

WHOLE HAND FRICTION I

③

Standing behind the receiver, support one side of their head and place your other hand above the opposite ear. Apply firm pressure to move the scalp up and down. Repeat on the other side.

RECEIVER'S SUPPORT
Use the forehead bracing technique to give the receiver support while applying strong strokes to the back of the head or neck. If you're left-handed, stand to the receiver's right shoulder and use your right hand for support while you work with your left.

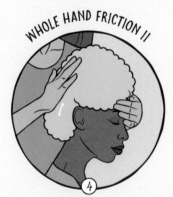

WHOLE HAND FRICTION II

④

Stand to one side of the receiver with one hand at the base of their skull. Apply firm pressure to move the scalp up and down. Repeat on the other side.

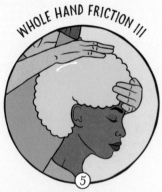

WHOLE HAND FRICTION III

⑤

Repeat the friction action on the top of the head.

RUFFLING

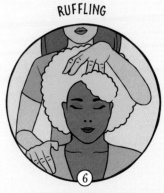

With one hand on the receiver's shoulder, use the fingers of the other hand to ruffle their hair, keeping light contact with the scalp. Toss long hair at the nape of the neck. Keep your touch light.

PLUCKING

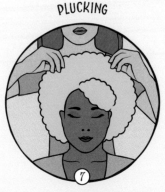

With your fingers long, land softly on the head and spring off quickly, bringing your fingers and thumbs together. Repeat this movement in different places until you've covered the entire scalp.

SCALP CHAMPI

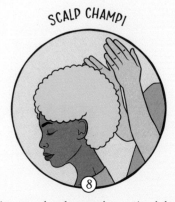

Bring your hands over the receiver's head, palms facing each other with fingers together. Alternate your hands to make quick, light hitting movements over the top of the head. Repeat the movement in different places until you've covered the entire scalp.

EAR SQUEEZE

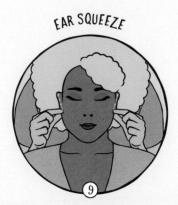

Squeeze the outer part of the ears using your forefingers and thumbs, starting at the earlobes and working up.

FOCUSED INDIAN HEAD MASSAGE RITUALS

EAR PULL

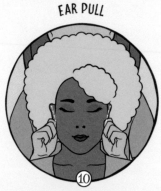

Using light pressure, slowly pull the ears up and down, starting at the earlobes and working up.

FINGERTIP FRICTIONS

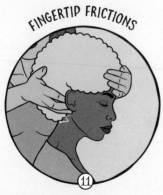

With the head tilted slightly forward in your hand, use your fingertips to apply friction in a zigzag motion along the base of the skull. Start behind the ear and move toward the midline, avoiding the spine. Switch hands and repeat on the other side.

HEEL RUB

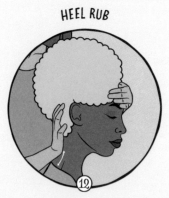

Still with one hand on the receiver's forehead, rub the base of the skull lightly and briskly with the heel and palm of the other hand in an up-and-down movement.

NECK OPENER

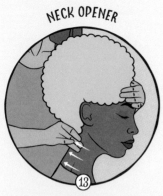

Bring your right hand to the top of the neck, grab the flesh there and pull it back. Grab at the middle of the neck and pull back again, then repeat at the base of the neck. Repeat the pulls a total of three times.

PALM ROLL

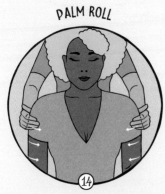

(14)

SHOULDER CHAMPI

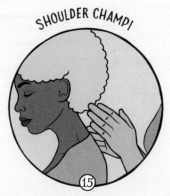

(15)

Place your hands on the receiver's upper arms, with your fingers in front and the base of your palms behind. With medium pressure, roll the palms forward over the muscles to meet your fingertips, being careful not to pinch the skin. Repeat in the middle of the upper arm, and then again just above the elbow. Repeat the whole process three times.

Bring your hands together in a prayer position. Keeping your wrists soft, make quick, light hitting movements with your pinky fingers across the receiver's shoulders. Focus on the muscles and avoid and bony prominences.

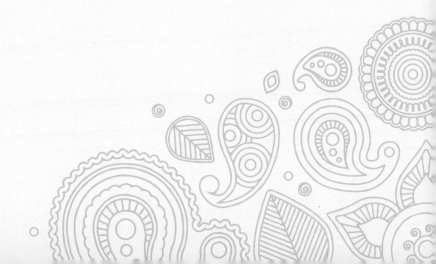

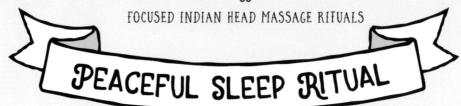

PEACEFUL SLEEP RITUAL

You can use this ritual to relieve stress and tension that can keep you from experiencing the benefits of nourishing and regenerative sleep. Use the breathing exercise, marma energy work, and massage techniques in a slow and meditative way to prepare for sleep.

The process

This ritual relieves restlessness and insomnia through guided breathwork, marma points stimulation that benefits deep sleep, and massage techniques designed to melt tension.

Marma points

You will be stimulating the Murdhi, Brahma Randra, Simanta, Shankha, and Ajna marma points (see pages 18–21). Stimulating the Murdhi point promotes restful sleep; massaging Brahma Randra can help with insomnia or irregular sleep; working the Simanta points is said to improve quality of relaxation; Shankha is calming and nourishing; and Ajna gives peace of mind.

Herbal oil recipe

After massaging you can apply the Peaceful Sleep Hair Oil (see page 39). You can also use a little oil on your fingers when stimulating the marma points.

Key massage strokes

EFFLEURAGE: PAGE 30
Circular; sweeping

PETRISSAGE: PAGE 30
Squeezing; shampooing; stroking; ironing

FRICTIONS: PAGE 31
Shearing; pulling

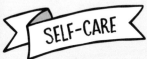

Alternate Hand Breathing

Sit in a straight-backed chair with the soles of your feet planted into the ground.
With your eyes closed, or open with a soft gaze, encourage your neck to rest in a
neutral position, and allow your jaw to relax. Notice your current breathing pattern
without changing it or making judgments.

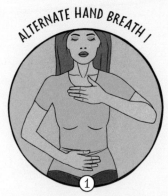

Place one hand on your belly and one on your
chest. Without changing your breathing,
notice which hand rises and falls with
the breath.

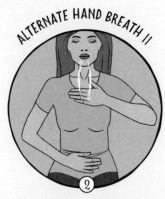

Now change your breathing to only breathe
into the hand on the chest. Bring your
awareness to how this feels. Continue for
at least three breaths.

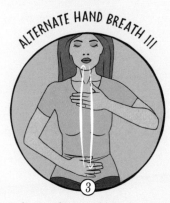

Switch your focus and breathe into the
hand on your belly only. Be aware of any
sensations. Continue for at least three breaths.

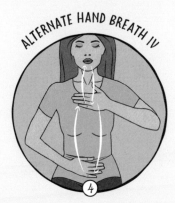

Now breathe in a wave-like fashion. Start by
breathing into the hand on the chest, then fill
the belly with air, allowing that hand to also
rise. Let the breath exhale from the belly, then
the chest. Repeat for at least three breaths.

Marma Sequence

Use your middle and ring fingers in slow, clockwise circles—seven is a good number, however if you are new to Ayurvedic head massage then three circles may be preferable. You can use a herbal oil for this sequence if you wish. Refer to pages 18–21 for guidance with locating the points.

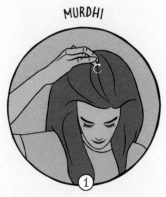

MURDHI

Locate the Murdhi marma point. Massage using light pressure, moving your fingers in slow, clockwise circles seven times.

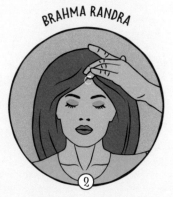

BRAHMA RANDRA

The Brahma Randra point is located at the center of the scalp just above the hairline. Massage this point using light pressure and seven slow, clockwise circles.

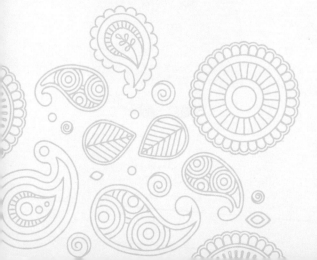

PEACEFUL SLEEP RITUAL

SIMANTA

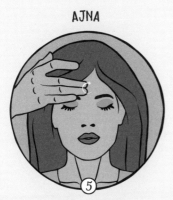

Locate the Simanta points across the summit of the skull and massage using light pressure, moving your fingers in slow, clockwise circles seven times.

SHANKHA

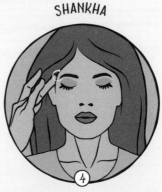

Locate the Shankha point in the hollows of the temples. Stimulate one side with seven clockwise circles. On the final repetition, leave your fingers on the temple and focus on feelings of sleepiness for three breaths. Repeat on the other side.

AJNA

Ajna is known as the third-eye point, and is found in the center of the forehead. Use your middle and ring fingers to make seven slow, clockwise circles.

Massage Sequence

Use slow movements and light pressure for a sedating effect
and to avoid energizing your body.

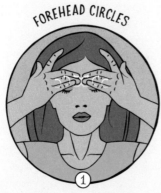

FOREHEAD CIRCLES

Place the middle and ring fingers of each hand
between the eyebrows. Make slow circles
using light pressure above the eyebrows,
traveling toward the outside of both brows.
Repeat seven times.

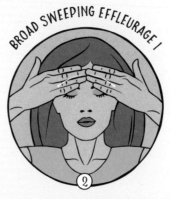

BROAD SWEEPING EFFLEURAGE I

Using both hands, sweep the forehead. Use
light pressure while slowly stroking out
toward the temples.

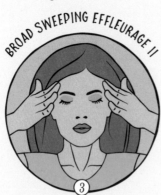

BROAD SWEEPING EFFLEURAGE II

Pause briefly to apply pressure at the temples.
Complete the whole Broad Sweeping
Effleurage sequence three times.

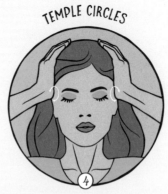

TEMPLE CIRCLES

Bring the base of your palms to the temples
and move both hands in slow, clockwise
circles, seven times in total.

TEMPLES SQUEEZE AND LIFT

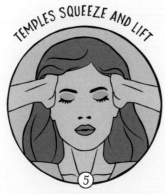

Bring the base of your palms to your temples.
Simultaneously squeeze and lift toward your
hairline, allowing the palms to drag the tissue
in a shearing movement. Repeat three times.

SHAMPOOING

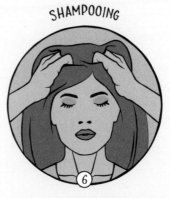

Make circular movements using the fingertips
and thumbs of both hands in a "shampoo-
like" motion all over the scalp.

SHOULDER SQUEEZE

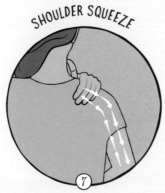

Use your left hand to gently squeeze the tissue
of your right shoulder near the neck. Repeat
at intervals moving along the shoulder and
down the upper arm to the elbow. Work back
up the arm in the same way. Make three
rounds and repeat on the other side.

SHOULDER SWEEP

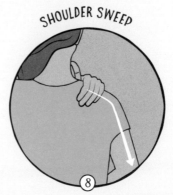

Use your left palm in one motion to slowly
sweep along your right shoulder, starting at
the base of your neck, moving out and down
the right arm. Do this three times, then repeat
using your right hand on your left shoulder.

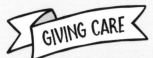
GIVING CARE

Marma Sequence

Verbally guide the receiver through the steps of the alternate hand breathing technique detailed on page 89. Use your middle and ring fingers in slow, clockwise circles—seven is a good number; however, if you are new to Ayurvedic head massage then three circles may be preferable. You can use a herbal oil for this sequence if you wish. Refer to pages 18–21 for guidance with locating the points.

MURDHI

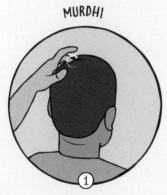

BRAHMA RANDRA

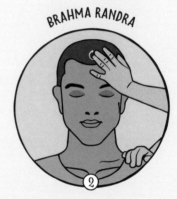

Standing behind the receiver, locate the Murdhi point with the middle and ring fingers and make seven slow, clockwise circles.

Locate the Brahma Randra marma at the center of the scalp just above the hairline and use light pressure with the middle and ring fingers to make seven slow, clockwise circles.

SIMANTA

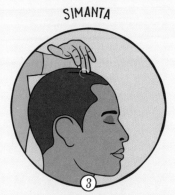

Locate the Simanta points across the summit
of the skull and massage using light pressure,
moving your fingers in slow, clockwise
circles seven times.

SHANKHA

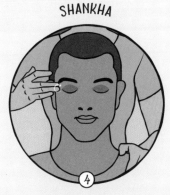

Locate the Shankha point in the hollows
of the temples. Stimulate one side with
seven clockwise circles, then repeat on
the other side.

AJNA

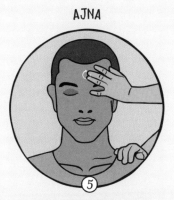

Ajna is known as the third eye-point, and is
found in the center of the forehead. Use your
middle and ring fingers to make seven slow,
clockwise circles.

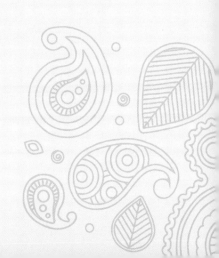

Massage Sequence

Stand behind the receiver with the palms of your hands on their forehead at the hairline, with fingers overlapping. Relax in this position to create a sense of calm and stillness. Use slow movements and light pressure for the massage.

STROKING

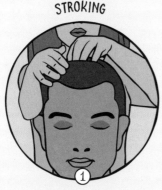

Bring one hand over the top of the head with your fingers pointing toward the hairline. Slowly rake through the hair, following with the other hand in a wave-like motion. Continue to the sides of the head, stopping at the ears. Repeat five to seven times.

FOREHEAD CIRCLES

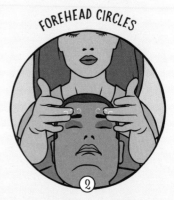

Stand behind the receiver and use a rolled towel to stabilize their head. Make small, slow circles using light pressure with the fingertips above the eyebrows. Start near the inner edge of the brows and work toward the outside edges. Repeat seven times.

BROAD SWEEPING EFFLEURAGE I

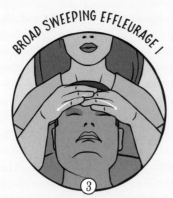

Using both hands, sweep the forehead. Use light pressure while slowly stroking out toward the temples.

BROAD SWEEPING EFFLEURAGE II

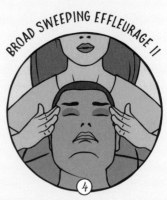

Pause briefly to apply pressure at the temples. Complete the whole Broad Sweeping Effleurage sequence three times.

TEMPLE CIRCLES

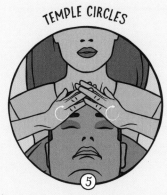

(5)

Bring the base of your palms to the temples
and make seven slow, clockwise circles.

TEMPLES SQUEEZE AND LIFT

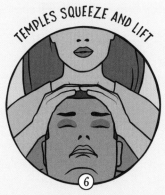

(6)

Still with the base of your palms on the
temples, gently squeeze and lift toward
the hairline.

TOWEL STABILIZING

The rolled-towel method of support is
useful when applying compressions and
frictions. Place a rolled towel on your
chest or belly and ask the receiver to lean
back onto it, so they don't strain their
neck muscles during the massage.

SHAMPOOING

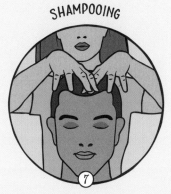

(7)

Use light pressure with the fingertips and
thumbs of both hands in a "shampoo-like"
motion all over the scalp.

NECK OPENER

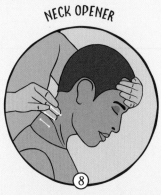

⑧

Stand at the receiver's left shoulder with your left hand cupping their forehead for support. Bring your right hand to the top of the neck, grab the flesh there and pull it back. Grab at the middle of the neck and pull back again, then repeat at the base of the neck. Repeat the sequence a total of three times.

IRONING DOWN I

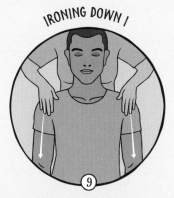

⑨

Standing behind the receiver again, use medium pressure with the palms and heels of your hands to compress the muscles from the top of the arms down to the elbows.

IRONING DOWN II

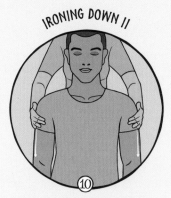

⑩

Use the same technique to compress down the sides of the arms.

IRONING DOWN III

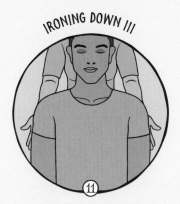

⑪

Finally, using light pressure, iron down the back of the arms. Repeat the whole Ironing Down sequence three times.

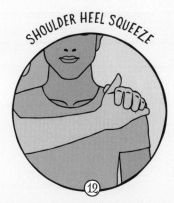

Stand at the receiver's left shoulder and reach across to their right shoulder, draping your right arm in front and left arm across their back. Using light pressure at first, and working to deeper pressure, squeeze the muscle on the top of the shoulder with the heels of your hands in several places. Switch sides to repeat on their left shoulder.

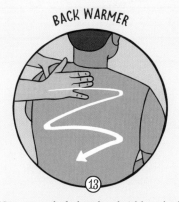

Use your whole hand to briskly rub all over the receiver's back.

GIVER'S COMFORT
Remember to keep your shoulders down and relaxed.

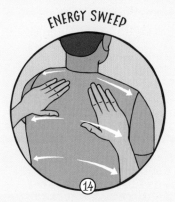

To bring a sense of closure to the massage, stand behind the receiver with loose hands positioned on the shoulders on either side of the spine. Sweep your hands out along the shoulders and off the body. Do the same on the upper back, and then the mid-back. Repeat three times in total.

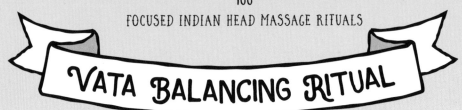

VATA BALANCING RITUAL

This is a slow and nourishing ritual to ground and balance excessive Vata energy, which can help bring you to a state of relaxed awareness and clarity of mind during busy times.

Consider warming your space and hair oil, as well as incorporating herbal heat packs to soothe Vata qualities. Vata can be very responsive to touch and may prefer light pressure, so always begin with a light touch and only work into stronger pressure if desired.

The process

For self-care, begin with a pranayama breathing exercise selected specifically for Vata dosha, or, when giving care, start with chakra balancing. Slow, intentional marma work and massage techniques complete the ritual.

Marma points

You will be stimulating the Brahma Randra, Avarta, and Utkshepa marma points (see pages 18–21). Brahma Randra is traditionally massaged in order to balance hormones and support sleep patterns and body weight. The Avarta point soothes excessive Vata energy, while stimulating the Utkshepa point helps to calm the mind.

Chakra balancing

The breathing technique and hand positions are intended to balance the crown and heart chakras (see pages 16–17).

Key massage strokes

EFFLEURAGE: PAGE 30

Circular; sweeping

PETRISSAGE: PAGE 30

Squeezing; shampooing; stroking

FRICTIONS: PAGE 31

Pulling

Herbal oil recipe

If you would like to use an oil for the massage, choose the Dosha Balancing Hair Oil (see page 39). You can also use a little oil on your fingers when stimulating the marma points.

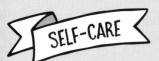

Bee Breath

The humming vibration created during bee breath calms the nervous system, massages the vagus nerve, and soothes anxious Vata. It's an excellent practice to help shake loose excess mental tension, allowing you to be present and focus inward.

INHALE

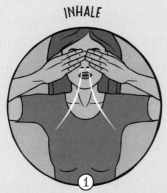

EXHALE

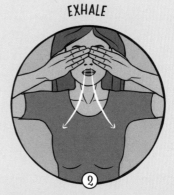

Lightly cover your eyes with your fingertips and use your thumbs to close your ears. Close your mouth and inhale through your nose, filling your lungs to capacity.

Slowly breathe out through your nose making a low humming sound in your throat until you've exhaled completely. Repeat the inhale and humming exhale at your own pace for two to three minutes.

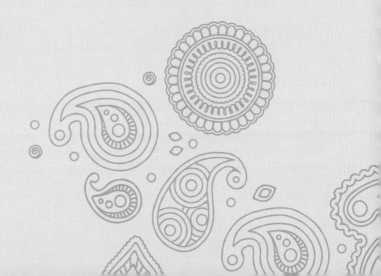

Marma Sequence

Use your middle and ring fingers in slow, counterclockwise circles—if you are new to Ayurvedic head massage you may prefer to make three, not seven, circles. Use a herbal oil if you wish. Refer to pages 18–21 for guidance with locating the points.

BRAHMA RANDRA

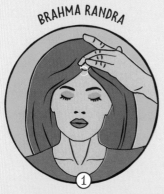

The Brahma Randra point is located at the center of the scalp just above the hairline. Massage this point using light pressure and seven slow, counterclockwise circles.

AVARTA

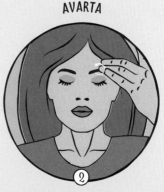

Avarta is found on the forehead, directly in the middle of each eyebrow. Massage using seven slow, counterclockwise circles.

UTKSHEPA

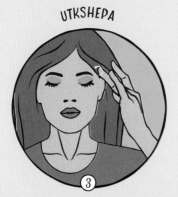

Locate Utkshepa on the side of the head, just above the ear on the temporal arteries. Massage using seven slow, counterclockwise circles. Repeat on the other side of the head with the other hand.

Massage Sequence

For this massage keep your movements slow and with a light touch.

SHOULDER SQUEEZE

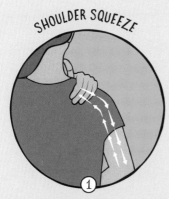

Use one hand to gently squeeze the tissue of the other shoulder, near the neck. Repeat at intervals down to the elbow and back up. After three rounds, repeat on the other arm.

JAWLINE SWEEP

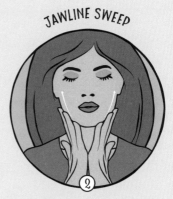

Bring your hands together in front of your chin, with fingers slightly open. Use slow, sweeping motions to follow the jawline up toward the ears. Repeat three times.

FOREHEAD CIRCLES

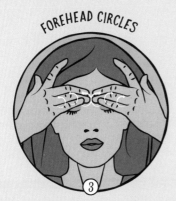

Place the middle and ring fingers of each hand between the eyebrows. Make slow circles using light pressure above the eyebrows, traveling toward the outer point of both brows. Repeat seven times.

SHAMPOOING AND STROKING

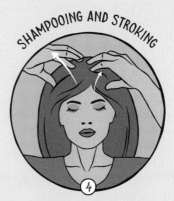

Use your fingertips to "shampoo" all over the scalp for a few minutes. Slowly stroke through your hair with alternate hands in a wave-like motion. Continue down the sides, stopping at the ears. Repeat five to seven times.

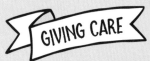

Chakra Balancing

Begin by bringing the palms of your hands to rest on the receiver's shoulders and ask them to take several deep breaths. Connect your breathing pattern to theirs and feel the ground under your feet. Create equal balance and pressure through the entire surface of the soles of your feet.

CROWN

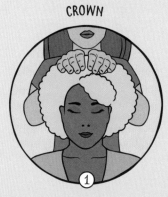

Bring the palms of your hands to rest on the crown of the receiver's head. Stay here for several breaths as you continue your balanced stance, opening the crown chakra.

HEART

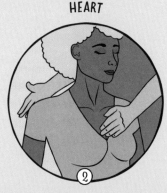

Stand to the receiver's left shoulder, bringing your left hand to hover over their upper chest, just below the collarbone. Bring your right hand to hover over the center of their upper back, between the shoulder blades. Remain here for several breaths.

AURA SWEEP

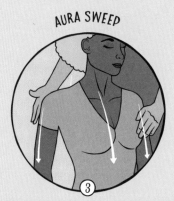

Close the chakra balancing ritual by hovering both hands several inches away from the receiver's body and sweeping them down the sides, front, and back of the body.

Marma Sequence

Use your middle and ring fingers in slow, counterclockwise circles—if you are new
to head massage you may prefer to make three, not seven, circles. Once you have
massaged each point as instructed, repeat the whole sequence twice more. Use a
herbal oil if you wish. Refer to pages 18–21 for guidance with locating the points.

BRAHMA RANDRA

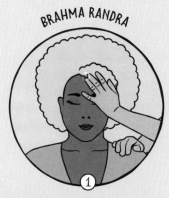

Locate Brahma Randra at the center of the
scalp just above the hairline and use light
pressure with the middle and ring fingers to
make seven slow, counterclockwise circles.

AVARTA

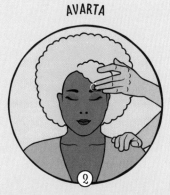

Place the non-working hand on the receiver's
shoulder for stability. The Avarta point is
found on the forehead, directly in the middle
of each eyebrow. Massage using seven slow,
counterclockwise circles.

UTKSHEPA

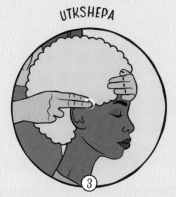

Locate Utkshepa on the side of the head, just
above the ears on the temporal arteries.
Massage using seven slow, counterclockwise
circles. Repeat on the other side of the head
with the other hand.

Massage Sequence

This massage will help the receiver to slow down and connect to the present when life seems hectic. Someone who shows more Vata-like characteristics can be very sensitive to touch. Work slowly and use light pressure, and check in with them to make sure they are completely comfortable.

SHOULDER SQUEEZE

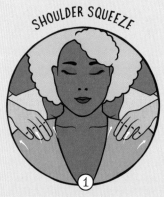

Place your hands on the outside edge of the shoulders with your fingers in front and thumbs behind. Squeeze the muscle on top of the shoulders with medium pressure. Hold for a few seconds, then release. Repeat at the middle of the shoulders, and again near the base of the neck. Make a total of three passes.

NECK OPENER

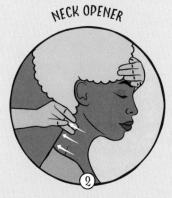

Stand at the receiver's left shoulder with your left hand cupping their forehead for support. Bring your right hand to the top of the neck, grab the flesh there and pull it back. Grab at the middle of the neck and pull back again, then repeat at the base of the neck. Repeat the sequence a total of three times.

FOREHEAD CIRCLES

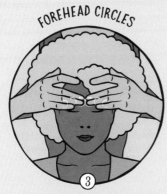

Make small, slow circles using light pressure with the fingertips above the eyebrows. Start near the inner edge of the brows and work toward the outside edges. Repeat seven times.

SHAMPOOING

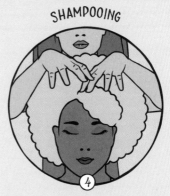

Use medium pressure with the fingertips and thumbs of both hands in a "shampoo-like" motion all over the scalp. Slowly shampoo for two to three minutes

STROKING

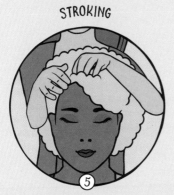

Bring one hand over the top of the head with your fingers pointing toward the hairline. Slowly rake through the hair, following with the other hand in a wave-like motion. Continue to the sides of the head, stopping at the ears. Repeat five to seven times.

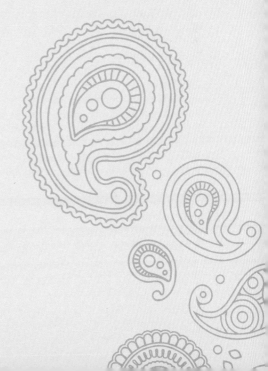

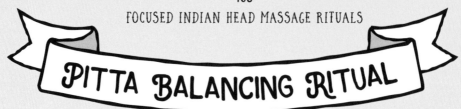

PITTA BALANCING RITUAL

This ritual was designed to cool and help balance the typically hot and sometimes impatient Pitta energy. Pittas enjoy honing-in on what's most important and getting the job done better than anyone else.

The most pleasing massage techniques for a Pitta type use an even and precise touch that moves outward, which encourages muscles and connective tissues to expand out into space.

The process

For self-care, begin with a pranayama breathing exercise selected specifically for Pitta dosha, or, when giving care, start with chakra balancing. Slow, intentional marma work and massage techniques complete the ritual.

Marma points

You will be stimulating the Shankha, Ajna, and Murdhi marma points (see pages 18–21). The Shankha point is emotionally nourishing and helps you to feel at peace. Ajna supports an energetic balance between the body, mind, and emotions, while Murdhi is traditionally stimulated to support healthy blood pressure.

Chakra balancing

The breathing technique and hand positions are intended to balance the third-eye and crown chakras (see pages 16–17).

Key massage strokes

EFFLEURAGE: PAGE 30
Circular; gliding; sweeping

PETRISSAGE: PAGE 30
Pinching; stroking; ironing; rolling

FRICTIONS: PAGE 31
Zigzags; tugging; pulling; superficial rubbing

Herbal oil recipe

If you would like to use an oil for the massage, choose the Dosha Balancing Hair Oil (see page 39). You can also use a little oil on your fingers when stimulating the marma points

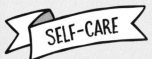

Cooling Breath

To pacify fiery Pitta energy and release feelings of irritation,
try this simple yet effective cooling breathing practice.

INHALE

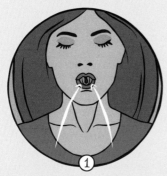

EXHALE

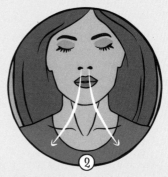

Stick out your tongue and curl the sides
inward in the shape of a tube or a straw.
Inhale by sucking air through your tongue,
filling your lungs to capacity while also
making a hissing sound.

Exhale evenly through both nostrils.
Repeat the inhale and exhale for two
to three minutes.

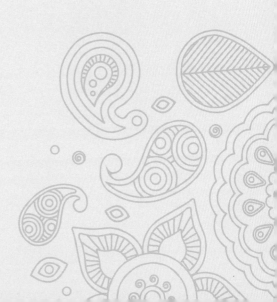

Marma Sequence

Use your middle and ring fingers in slow, counterclockwise circles—you may prefer to make three, not seven, circles. Massage each point then repeat the whole sequence twice more. Refer to pages 18–21 for guidance with locating the points.

SHANKHA

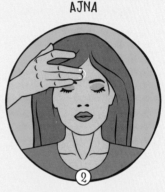

AJNA

Locate the Shankha point in the hollows of the temples. Stimulate one side with seven counterclockwise circles, then repeat on the other side.

Ajna is known as the third-eye point, and is found in the center of the forehead. Use your middle and ring fingers to make seven slow, counterclockwise circles.

MURDHI

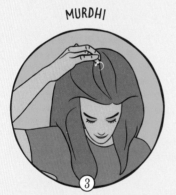

Locate the Murdhi marma. Massage the point using light pressure, moving your fingers in seven slow, counterclockwise circles. Repeat the whole sequence in order twice more.

Massage Sequence

Use these techniques to support yourself through times of stress. Pitta dosha types respond to an even and precise touch that expands tissues outward.

NECK OPENER

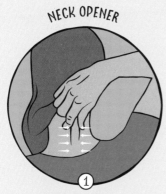

Squeeze the back of the neck with the right hand at intervals, starting from the top of the neck and moving down. Repeat with the left hand.

BROW BONE PINCH

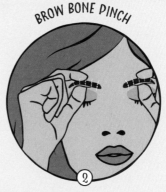

Beginning close to the nose, lightly pinch the eyebrows all along the brow bone between the thumbs and forefingers. Complete three passes in total.

FOREHEAD GLIDES

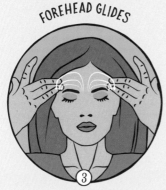

Place the middle and ring fingers of each hand between the eyebrows. Using gentle pressure, glide the fingers straight up and out to follow your hairline. Repeat the action midway between your hairline and eyebrow, and once more right above the eyebrows. Complete the sequence three times in total.

VERTICAL ZIGZAGS

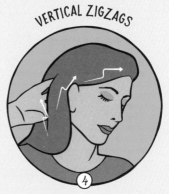

Make short, quick zigzag movements with the fingertips of one hand on the same side of the scalp. Working upward each time, start along your hairline to the temples, repeat behind the ear, and again at the back of the head. Switch hands to massage the other side of the head.

HAIR TUGGING

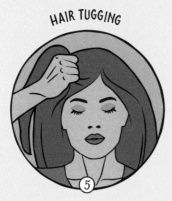

Using one hand at a time, grab fistfuls of hair at the scalp and quickly tug the hair in an upward motion at the roots. Repeat in several places all over the scalp.

STROKING

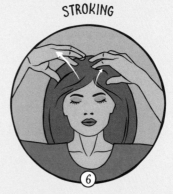

Beginning from the top of the head at the hairline, slowly stroke through your hair with alternate hands in a wave-like motion. Continue down the sides of the head, stopping at the ears. Repeat five to seven times.

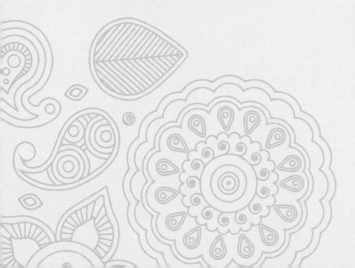

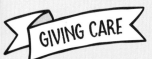
GIVING CARE

Chakra Balancing

Begin by bringing the palms of your hands to rest on the receiver's shoulders and ask them to take several deep breaths. Connect your breathing pattern to theirs and feel the ground under your feet. Create equal balance and pressure through the entire surface of the soles of your feet.

THIRD EYE

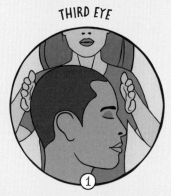

Bring the palms of your hands to hover one in front of the receiver's forehead and one behind their head in line with the third-eye chakra. Stay here for several breaths.

CROWN

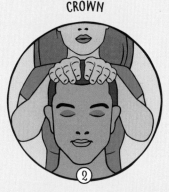

Bring the palms of your hands to rest on the crown of the receiver's head. Stay here for several breaths as you continue your balanced stance, opening the crown chakra.

AURA SWEEP

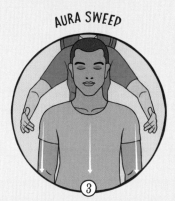

Close the chakra balancing ritual by hovering both hands several inches away from the receiver's body and sweeping them down the sides, front, and back of the body.

Marma Sequence

Use your middle and ring fingers in slow, counterclockwise circles—if you are new to head massage you may prefer to make three, not seven, circles. Once you have massaged each point as instructed, repeat the whole sequence twice more. You can use a herbal oil if you wish. Refer to pages 18–21 for guidance with locating points.

SHANKHA

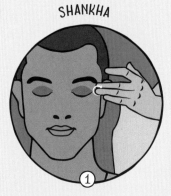

Locate the Shankha point in the hollows of the temples. Stimulate one side with seven slow, counterclockwise circles, then repeat on the other side.

AJNA

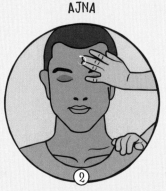

Ajna is known as the third eye-point, and is found in the center of the forehead. Use your middle and ring fingers to make seven slow, counterclockwise circles.

MURDHI

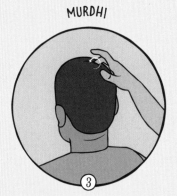

Standing behind the receiver, locate the Murdhi point with the middle and ring fingers and make seven slow, counterclockwise circles. Repeat the whole sequence in order twice more.

PITTA BALANCING RITUAL

Massage Sequence

Pitta dosha types enjoy even and precise touch that expands tissues outward.

IRONING OUT I

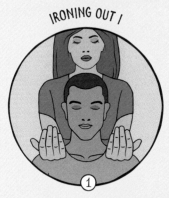

Place your forearms on each shoulder near the base of the neck. With your hands slightly higher than your elbows, turn your palms to face the sky.

IRONING OUT II

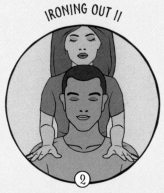

Using firm to medium pressure, slide both forearms simultaneously across the top of the shoulders, twisting your arms so the palms face the ground as you come to the end of the movement. Complete the whole Ironing Out sequence a total of three times.

GIVER'S COMFORT
Remember to keep your shoulders down and relaxed.

PALM ROLL

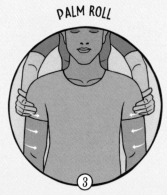

NECK OPENER

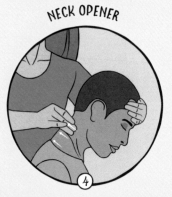

Place your hands on the receiver's upper arms, with your fingers in front and the base of your palms behind. With medium pressure, roll the palms forward over the muscles to meet your fingertips, being careful not to pinch the skin. Repeat in the middle of the upper arm, and then again just above the elbow. Repeat the whole process three times.

Stand at the receiver's left shoulder. Use your left hand to cup their forehead for support. Tilt the head forward into your hand slightly. Bring your right hand to the top of the neck, grab the flesh there and pull it back. Grab at the middle of the neck and pull back again, then repeat at the base of the neck. Repeat the entire sequence a total of three times.

RECEIVER'S SUPPORT

Use the forehead bracing technique to give the receiver support while applying strong strokes to the back of the neck. If you're left-handed, stand to the receiver's right shoulder and use your right hand for support while you work with your left.

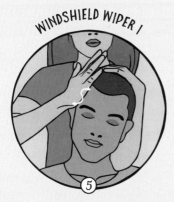

WINDSHIELD WIPER I

(5)

Stand behind the receiver and support one
side of their head using the bracing technique.
Use the heel of the other hand to lightly rub
over one side of the head, moving your hand
from side to side like a windshield wiper.

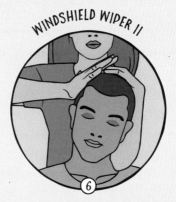

WINDSHIELD WIPER II

(6)

Next, use your whole hand to ruffle the top
of the receiver's head. Repeat the whole
Windshield Wiper technique on the other side
of the head, then continue with two more
rounds, alternating between each side.

BRACING

The neck bracing technique will provide
support for the receiver during frictions.
Stand behind the receiver and bend one
arm at the elbow. Place the bent arm on
the receiver's shoulder and lightly lean
their head into the palm of your hand to
offer support while working on the
opposite side of the head.

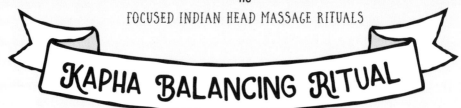

KAPHA BALANCING RITUAL

This energetic ritual will enliven the Kapha dosha. Kapha types tend to struggle with sluggish energy when they're out of balance, and enjoy movement that's fresh and dynamic to get them out of a slump.

Kapha types love creativity, so don't be afraid to use your imagination to combine and create energetic movements that you know they'll like.

The process

For self-care, begin with a pranayama breathing exercise selected specifically for Kapha dosha, or, when giving care, start with chakra balancing. Three marma points are then stimulated, followed by a vigorous massage to complete the ritual.

Marma points

You will be stimulating the Kathanadi, Arshak, and Manya marma points (see pages 18–21). The Kathanadi point supports healthy circulation and moves congestion. Arshak and Manya both support lymphatic drainage, while Manya also moves congestion.

Chakra balancing

The breathing technique and hand positions are intended to balance the throat and third-eye chakras (see pages 16–17), to help Kapha types stay open and connected to their truth.

Key massage strokes

EFFLEURAGE: PAGE 30

Circular; sweeping

PETRISSAGE: PAGE 30

Squeezing; stroking

FRICTIONS: PAGE 31

Shearing; superficial rubbing; zigzags; plucking; ruffling; pulling

Herbal oil recipe

If you would like to use an oil for the massage, choose the Dosha Balancing Hair Oil (see page 39). You can also use a little oil on your fingers when stimulating the marma points.

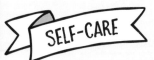
SELF-CARE

Bellows Breath

You can use the bellows breath to bring warmth to your body, stimulate digestion, improve your appetite, and fire up your metabolism.

Start this practice very slowly and mindfully at the rate of one breath per second. Limit yourself to three rounds of seven to ten breaths, taking a few relaxed breaths between each round. When you can speed it up without losing the evenness of your breath or the force, try working up to two breaths per second and 12 breaths per round. You'll find that your stamina will increase with practice.

EXHALE

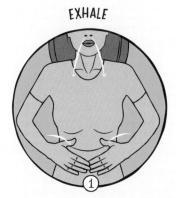

Exhale forcefully and audibly through your nose as you quickly contract your abdominal muscles.

INHALE

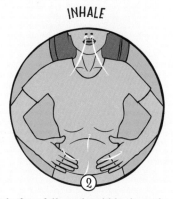

Inhale forcefully and audibly through your nose, allowing your belly to expand completely. Aim to make the inhalation and exhalation equal in timing and force.

SAFETY

Do not practice bellows breath after meals, during pregnancy, or if you have high blood pressure, a heart condition, or panic or anxiety issues.

TECHNIQUE PRACTICE

Try to coordinate the diaphragm and abdominal muscles so the air moves in and out of the lungs quickly. Bellows breath is a practice, so be patient with yourself as you learn to coordinate these movements.

Marma Sequence

Use your middle and ring fingers in slow, counterclockwise circles—if you are new to head massage you may prefer to make three, not seven, circles. Once you have massaged each point as instructed, repeat the whole sequence twice more. Use a herbal oil if you wish. Refer to pages 18–21 for guidance with locating the points.

KATHANADI

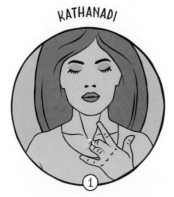

The Kathanadi points are located on both sides of the inside of the sternum's hollow notch. Make seven counterclockwise circles on one side and repeat on the other side.

ARSHAK

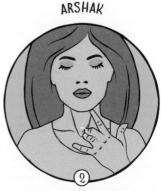

The Arshak points are located on each side of your body, just above the clavicle. Stimulate one side with seven slow, counterclockwise circles and repeat on the other side.

MANYA

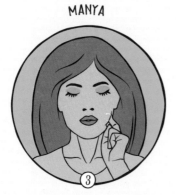

Locate the Manya point, four finger-widths below the earlobe. Stimulate one side with seven slow, counterclockwise circles and repeat on the other side. Repeat the whole sequence in order twice more.

Massage Sequence

A vigorous massage will focus your mind, move extra fluid
through your lymphatic system, and help break up congestion.

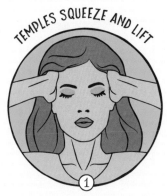

TEMPLES SQUEEZE AND LIFT

①

Bring the base of your palms to your temples.
Simultaneously squeeze and lift toward your
hairline, allowing the palms to drag the tissue
in a shearing movement. Repeat three times.

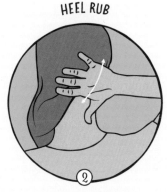

HEEL RUB

②

Rub the base of the skull lightly and briskly
with the heel of one hand in an up-and-down
movement. Use your right hand on the right
side and left hand for the left side.

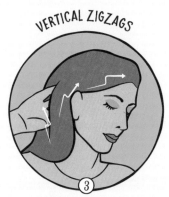

VERTICAL ZIGZAGS

③

Make short, quick zigzag movements with the
fingertips of one hand on the same side of the
scalp. Work upward along your hairline to the
temples, then repeat behind the ear and again
at the back of the head. Use the other hand
for the other side of the scalp.

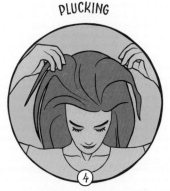

PLUCKING

④

With your fingers long, land softly on the
head and spring off quickly, bringing your
fingers and thumbs together. Repeat this
movement in different places until you've
covered your entire scalp.

RUFFLING

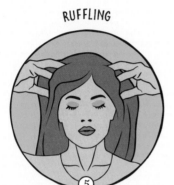

Using the fingers of both hands, briskly ruffle your hair keeping light contact with the scalp. Toss and flick long hair at the nape of the neck. Keep your touch light.

STROKING

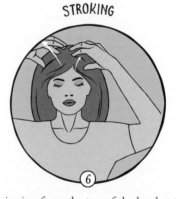

Beginning from the top of the head at the hairline, slowly stroke through your hair with alternate hands in a wave-like motion. Continue down the sides of the head, stopping at the ears. Repeat five to seven times.

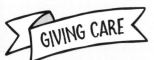

Chakra Balancing

Begin by bringing the palms of your hands to rest on the receiver's shoulders and ask them to take several deep breaths. Connect your breathing pattern to theirs and feel the ground under your feet. Create equal balance and pressure through the entire surface of the soles of your feet.

THROAT

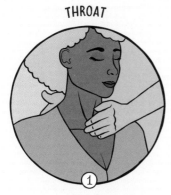

Standing to the receiver's left shoulder, bring the palm of your left hand to hover in front of the receiver's throat and the palm of the right hand to hover behind their neck. Stay here for several breaths.

THIRD EYE

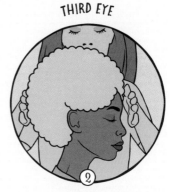

Bring the palms of your hands to hover one in front of the receiver's forehead and one behind their head in line with the third-eye chakra. Stay here for several breaths.

AURA SWEEP

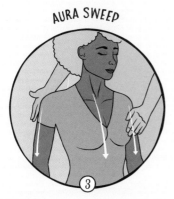

Close the chakra balancing ritual by hovering both hands several inches away from the receiver's body and sweeping them down the sides, front, and back of the body.

Marma Sequence

Use your middle and ring fingers in slow, counterclockwise circles—if you are new to Ayurvedic head massage you may prefer to make three, not seven, circles. Once you have massaged each point, repeat the whole sequence twice more. Use a herbal oil if you wish. Refer to pages 18–21 for guidance with locating the points.

KATHANADI

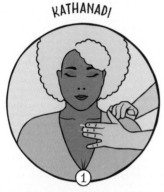

The Kathanadi points are located on both sides of the inside of the sternum's hollow notch. Stimulate each side with seven slow, counterclockwise circles.

ARSHAK

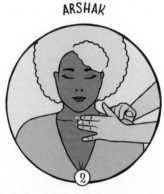

The Arshak points are located on each side of your body, just above the clavicle. Stimulate one side with seven slow, counterclockwise circles and repeat on the other side.

MANYA

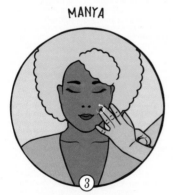

Locate the Manya point, four finger widths below the earlobe. Stimulate one side with seven slow, counterclockwise circles and repeat on the other side. Repeat the whole sequence in order twice more.

Massage Sequence

This is a lively massage sequence to help the receiver feel revitalized.

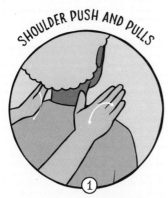

SHOULDER PUSH AND PULLS

①

Stand behind the receiver. Place the base of each palm at the top of each shoulder blade. Using medium pressure, push the muscles forward with your palm, moving up and over. Pull the muscles back by dragging your fingers toward you. Repeat three times.

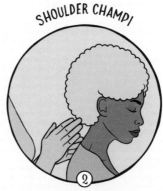

SHOULDER CHAMPI

②

Bring your hands together in a prayer position. Keeping your wrists soft, make quick, light hitting movements with your pinky fingers across the receiver's shoulders. Focus on the muscles and avoid any bony prominences.

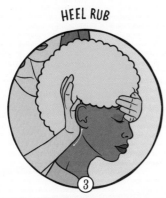

HEEL RUB

③

With one hand on the receiver's forehead, tilt the head slightly forward. Rub the base of the skull lightly and briskly with the heel and palm of the other hand in an up-and-down movement.

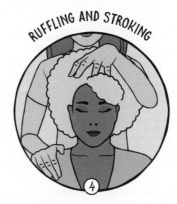

RUFFLING AND STROKING

④

With one hand on the receiver's shoulder, use the fingers of the other hand to ruffle their hair, keeping light contact with the scalp. Finish by Stroking (see page 107).

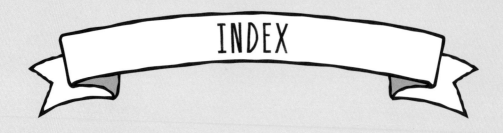

INDEX